seventeen

presents...

500
style tips

For *Seventeen*: writer, Emmy Favilla; designer: Wendy Robison; photo editor, Alana Anesh.

Seventeen 500 Style Tips

Library of Congress Cataloging-in-Publication Data

Favilla, Emmy.
  Seventeen presents 500 style tips : what to wear for school, weekend, parties & more! / Emmy Favilla.
      p. cm.
  Includes index.
  ISBN-13: 978-1-58816-641-8
  ISBN-10: 1-58816-641-4
  1. Girls' clothing. 2. Teenage girls—Clothing. 3. Fashion.
I. Seventeen. II. Title. III. Title: Seventeen presents five hundred style tips.
   TT562.F38 2007
   746.9'20835--dc22

                                        2007014623

10 9 8 7 6 5 4 3 2 1

Seventeen and Hearst Books are trademarks of Hearst Communications, Inc.

www.seventeen.com

For information about custom editions, special sales, premium and corporate purchases, please contact Sterling Sales Department at 800-805-5489 or specialsales@sterlingpub.com.

Distributed in Canada by Sterling Publishing
C/o Canadian Manda Group, 165 Dufferin Street
Toronto, Ontario, Canada M6K 3H6

Distributed in Australia by Capricorn Link (Australia) Pty. Ltd., P.O. Box 704, Windsor, NSW 2756 Australia
Printed in China

Sterling ISBN-13: 978-1-58816-641-8
          ISBN-10: 1-58816-641-4

seventeen
presents...

500
style tips

What to Wear for
School, Weekend, Parties & More!

HEARST BOOKS
A division of Sterling Publishing Co., Inc.

New York / London
www.sterlingpublishing.com

contents

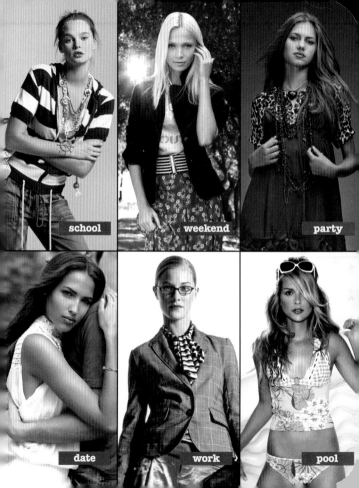

school

weekend

party

date

work

pool

hey!

No more stressing in front of the **closet**, debating what to wear! Consider *us* your personal **stylists**. This helpful book is jam-packed with cute outfit ideas and **quick** fashion tips—so you're sure to be the best **dressed** girl at *every* event.

–the editors of seventeen

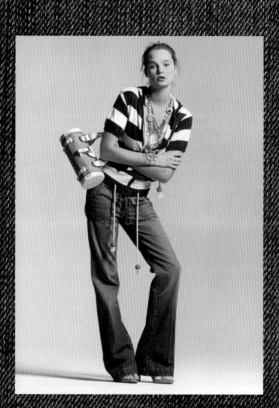

school

Rocker or retro, sporty or preppy—no matter what your style, you want to feel pretty and look great. Use the ideas in this section for cute school-appropriate styles—so you can feel confident whether you're taking notes *or* sitting at lunch with your friends!

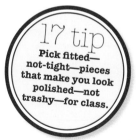

17 tip

Pick fitted—not-tight—pieces that make you look polished—not trashy—for class.

#1
wide-legged pants

do double duty: they add the look of curves to slim legs and thighs, and they balance a curvy tummy and hips.

great for all body types!

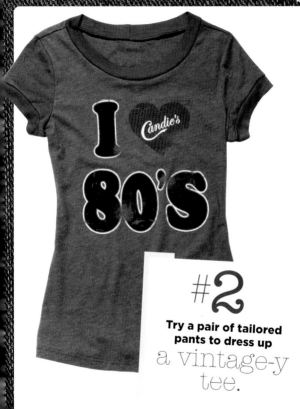

I ♥ Candie's 80'S

#2

Try a pair of tailored pants to dress up a vintage-y tee.

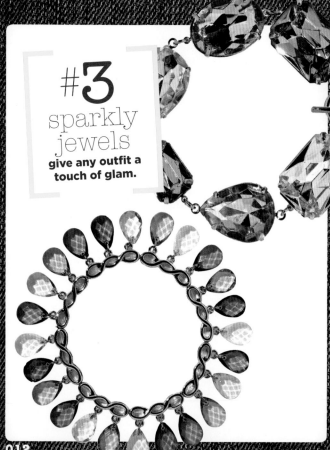

#3
sparkly jewels
give any outfit a touch of glam.

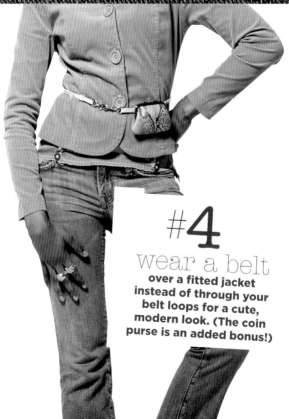

#4

wear a belt

over a fitted jacket instead of through your belt loops for a cute, modern look. (The coin purse is an added bonus!)

#5
layer a track jacket
under your blazer for a unique look!

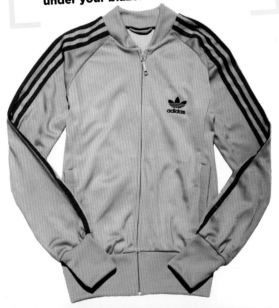

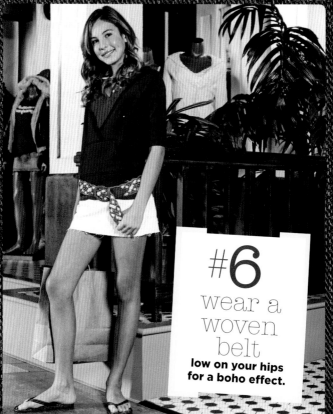

#6
wear a
woven
belt
**low on your hips
for a boho effect.**

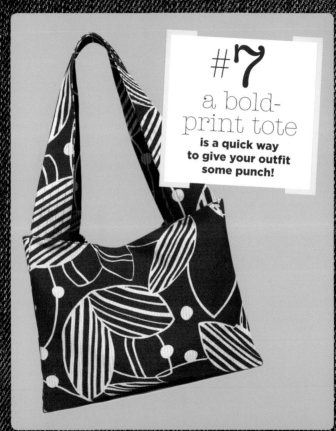

#7
a bold-print tote
is a quick way to give your outfit some punch!

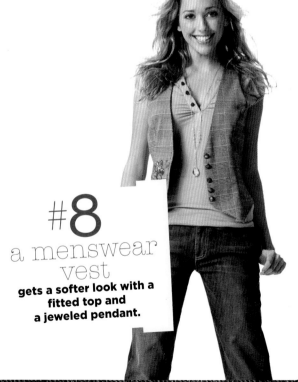

#8
a menswear vest
**gets a softer look with a
fitted top and
a jeweled pendant.**

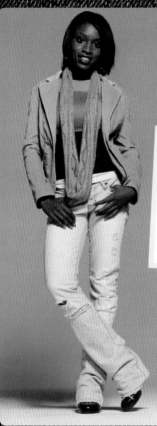

#9
a tailored blazer
instantly dresses up those edgy jeans.

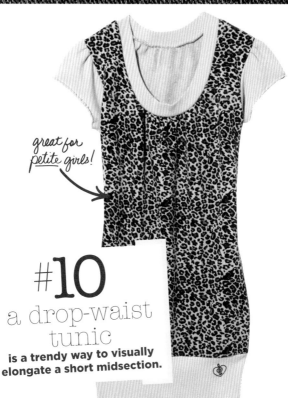

great for petite girls!

#10
a drop-waist tunic
is a trendy way to visually elongate a short midsection.

#11

super-
skinny
jeans

**look great under
longer tops so
you show off your
shape without
revealing too much.**

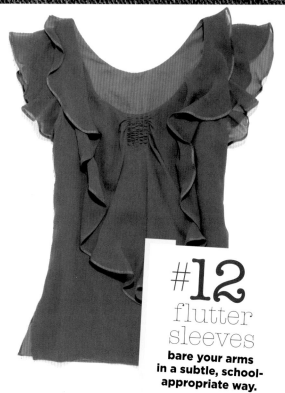

#12
flutter sleeves
bare your arms in a subtle, school-appropriate way.

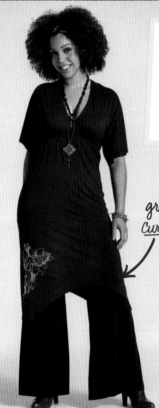

#13
a dress
**over wide-leg pants
streamlines hips.**

*great for
<u>Curvy thighs!</u>*

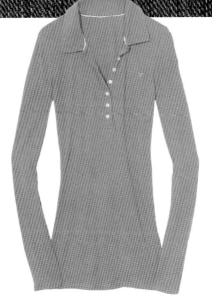

#14
a button-down polo
**is great for layering over a
cami or under a sweater—or both!**

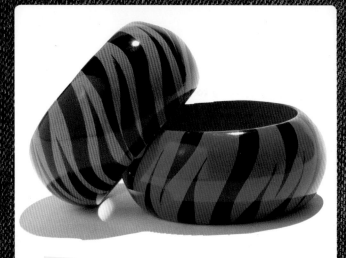

#15

pile on the bangles

to make any outfit a little bit funkier!

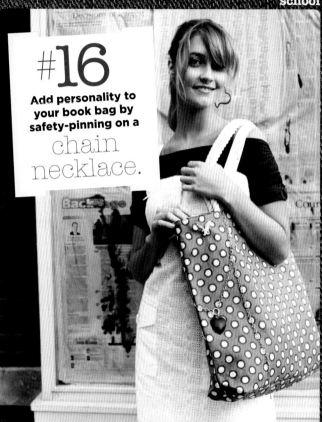

#16

Add personality to your book bag by safety-pinning on a

chain necklace.

#17

Give a layered tunic a more form-fitting shape with a low-slung belt.

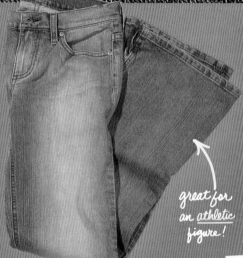

great for an athletic figure!

#18

faded jeans that are lighter
in front and darker on the sides slim fuller legs.

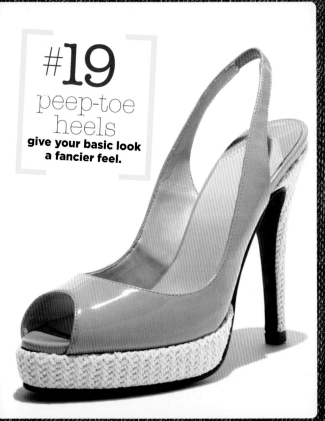

#19
peep-toe heels
give your basic look a fancier feel.

#20
a trapeze jacket

looks as polished as a blazer but has a flirtier vibe.

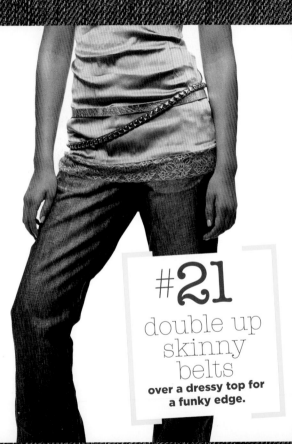

#21

double up
skinny
belts

**over a dressy top for
a funky edge.**

#22
a guy's tie
works great as a cool belt.

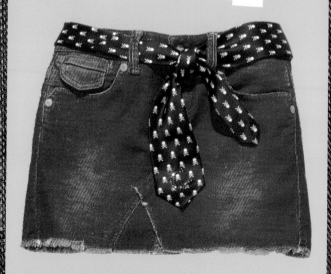

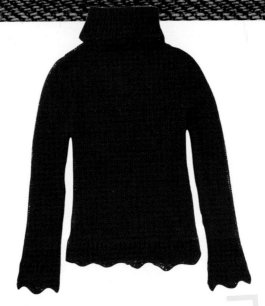

#23
layer a turtleneck
under your favorite spring dress—and you can wear it throughout the winter, too!

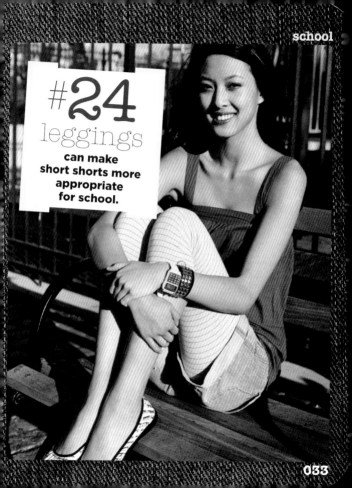

#24
leggings

can make short shorts more appropriate for school.

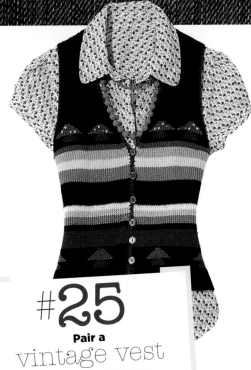

#25

Pair a

vintage vest

**with a printed blouse;
the two quirky pieces will work
together perfectly.**

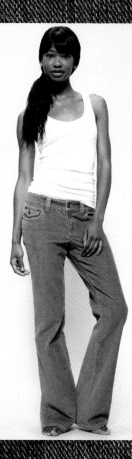

#26

boot-cut cords

**are more polished
than jeans
but still look chic.**

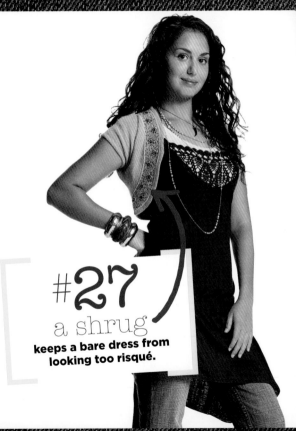

#27

a shrug

keeps a bare dress from looking too risqué.

#28
wear flat shoes

with skinny jeans in the spring, then swap them for tall boots in the fall.

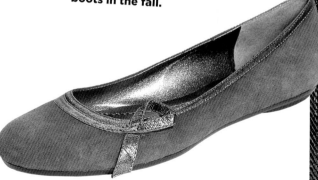

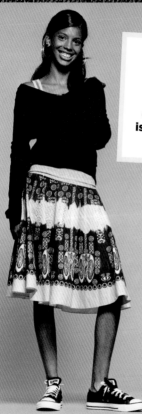

#29

a full skirt

is a classy way to girl-ify your sneakers.

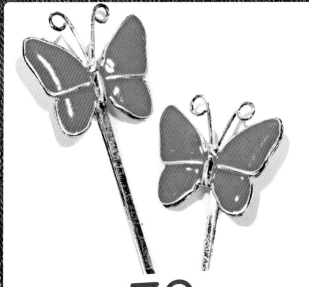

#30

funky hair accessories

give *any* look an eclectic edge.

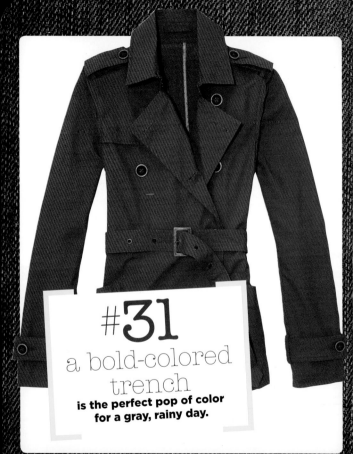

#31
a bold-colored trench
is the perfect pop of color for a gray, rainy day.

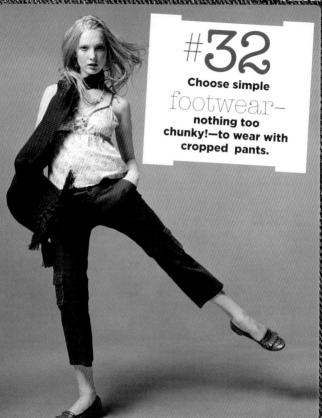

#32

Choose simple footwear— **nothing too chunky!—to wear with cropped pants.**

#33
capris
show off great calves (without being too clingy!).

great for curvy thighs!

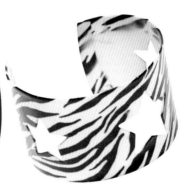

#34
zebra print pieces
have a cool rocker feel—but only wear one at a time!

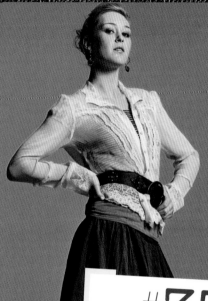

#35

be unexpected:
**wear a studded
belt with a delicate blouse.**

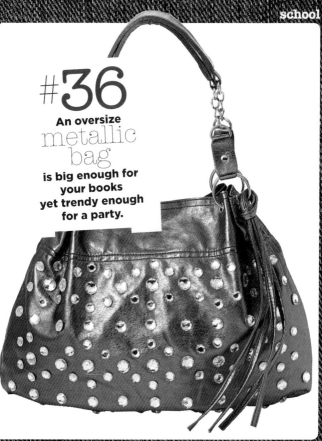

#36

An oversize
metallic
bag
**is big enough for
your books
yet trendy enough
for a party.**

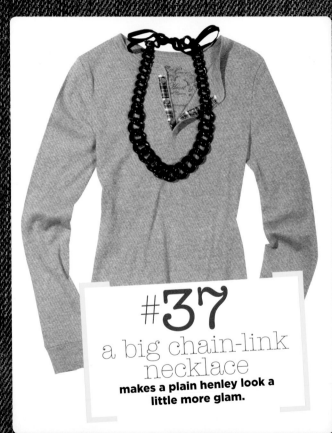

#37
a big chain-link necklace
makes a plain henley look a little more glam.

#38
layer a bright tank
under a striped top for an unexpected twist on a nautical vibe.

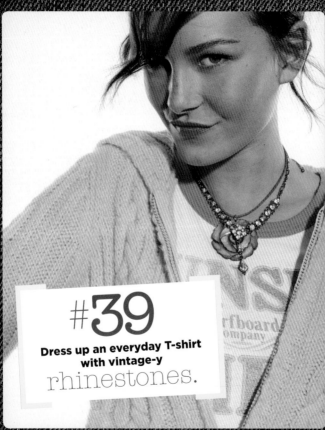

#39

Dress up an everyday T-shirt with vintage-y
rhinestones.

#40
a cropped jacket
is perfect for layering!

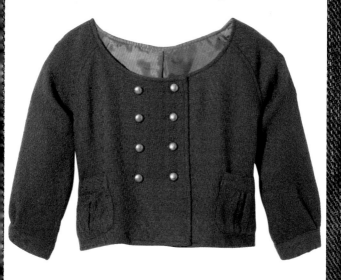

#41
drop pleats
look schoolgirl chic *and* don't add bulk to your middle.

great for <u>curvy</u> hips!

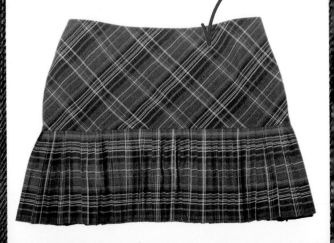

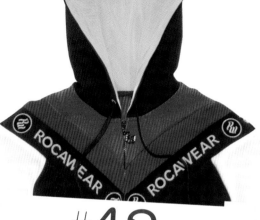

#42

mix a sporty jacket

**with more girly pieces
to get a flirty, unique style.**

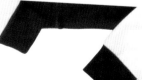

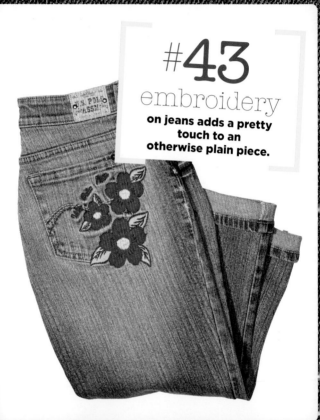

#43
embroidery

**on jeans adds a pretty
touch to an
otherwise plain piece.**

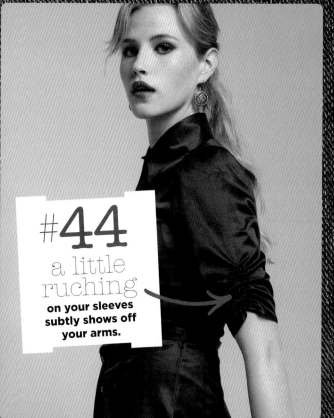

#44

a little ruching

on your sleeves subtly shows off your arms.

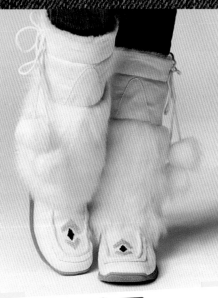

#45

wear furry boots

**with jeans and a cropped jacket
for a snow-bunny effect!**

#46

Dress up any pair of jeans by adding a

a belt with a
big buckle.

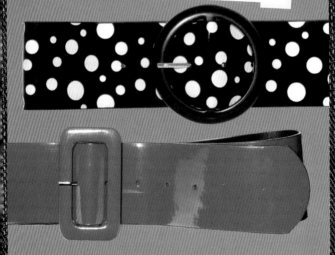

#47

Try an

argyle sweater

in candy-sweet colors for a modern preppy look.

#48

Wear a long-sleeve top under a

slip dress

so you can wear it on cool days.

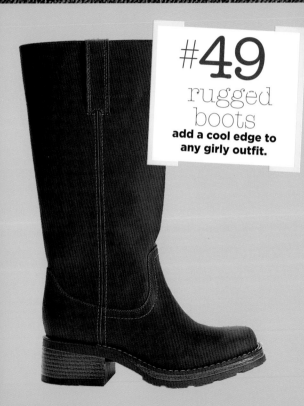

#49

rugged
boots
**add a cool edge to
any girly outfit.**

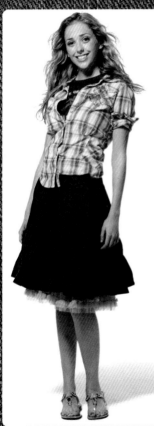

#50

Wear a frilly skirt to school with confidence— a plaid top **will dress it down just enough!**

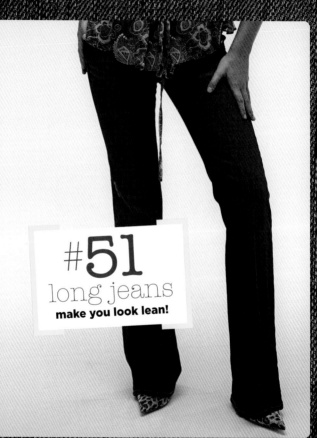

#51
long jeans
make you look lean!

#52
Recycle your mom's old
vintage scarves
and use them as fabulous headbands!

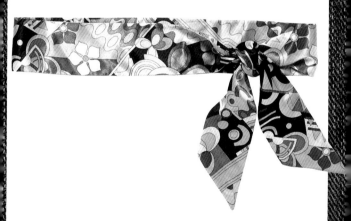

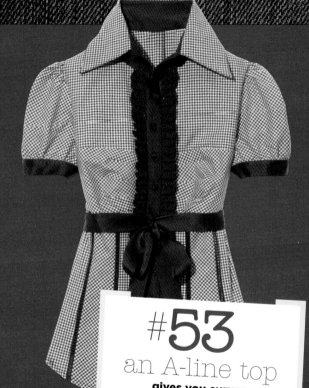

#53

an A-line top

**gives you curves
in all the right places.**

#54

a patent-
leather bag

takes a basic blouse and jeans up a notch.

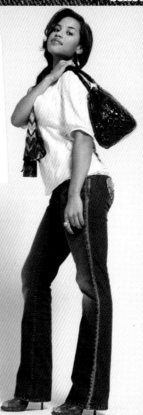

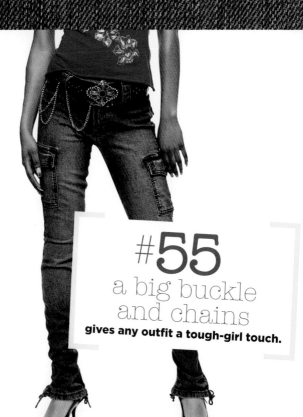

#55
a big buckle and chains
gives any outfit a tough-girl touch.

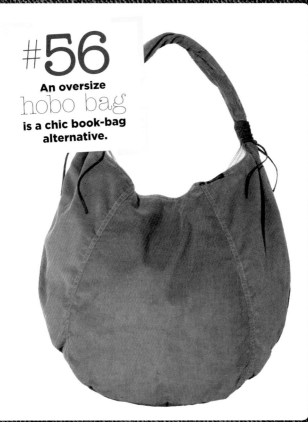

#56

An oversize
hobo bag
**is a chic book-bag
alternative.**

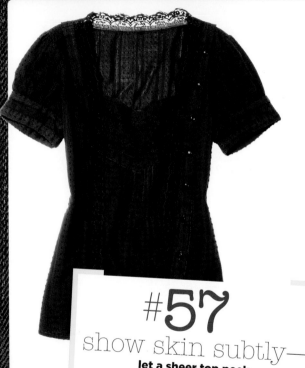

#57

show skin subtly—

**let a sheer top peek
out from under a cute jacket.**

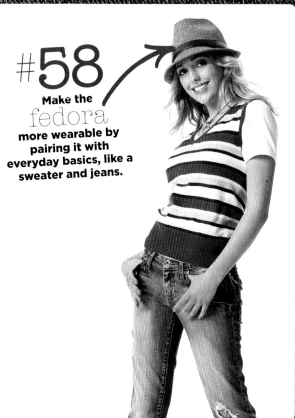

#58

Make the

fedora

more wearable by
pairing it with
everyday basics, like a
sweater and jeans.

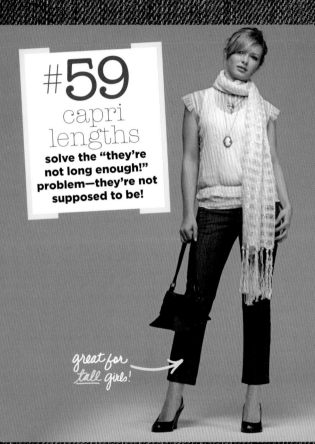

#59
capri lengths

solve the "they're not long enough!" problem—they're not supposed to be!

great for tall girls!

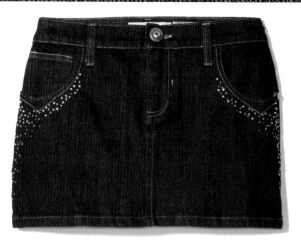

#60
rhinestones
**give a basic mini a little flash—
so you *really* stand out in
the hallways. But wear it with dark
tights when you're at school!**

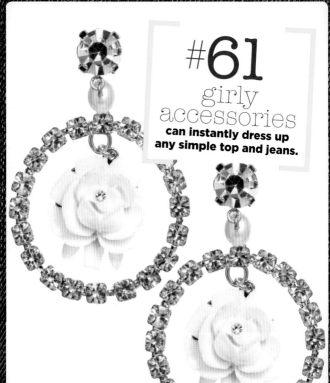

#61
girly
accessories
**can instantly dress up
any simple top and jeans.**

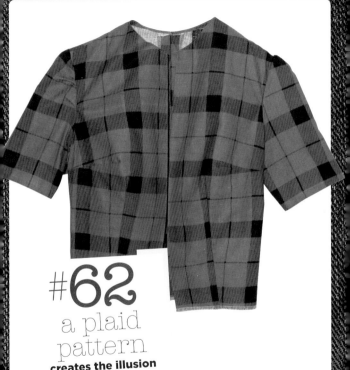

#62

a plaid
pattern

**creates the illusion
of curves.**

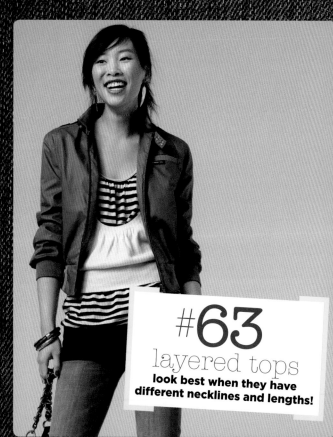

#63
layered tops
**look best when they have
different necklines and lengths!**

#64

Try cute

sneaker
flats

**to make a dress
casual enough for
school.**

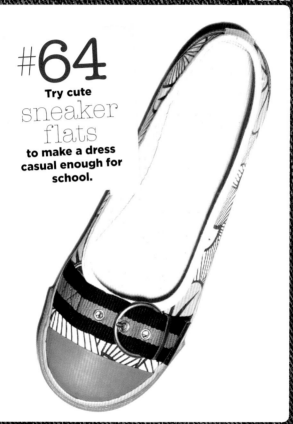

#65

epaulets

have a trendy military look *and* visually broaden shoulders.

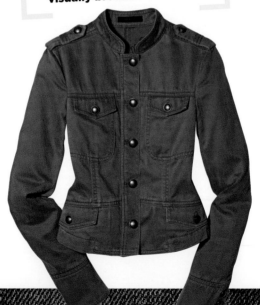

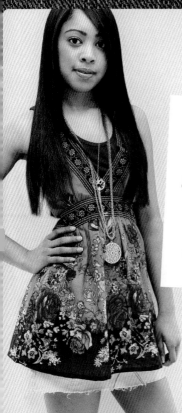

#66

Balance

a delicate peasant piece

with an unexpected, funky touch of denim.

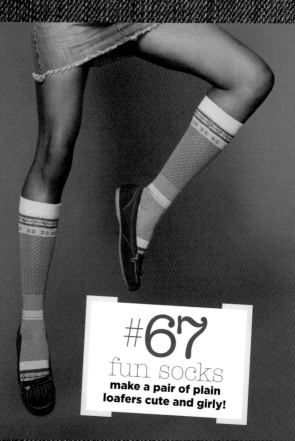

#67

fun socks

make a pair of plain loafers cute and girly!

#68

pair a loose-fitting top
with sleek pants so you don't look shapeless.

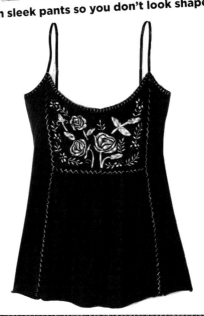

#69
pin a vintage-y brooch
in an unexpected spot to make a plain top special.

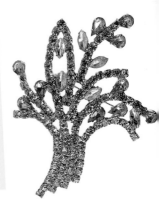

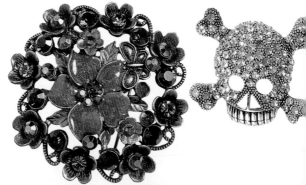

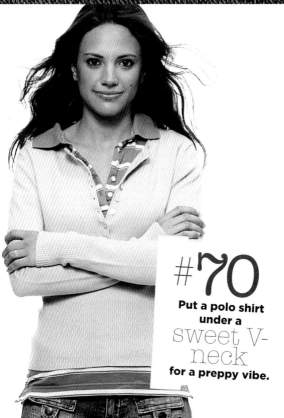

#70

**Put a polo shirt
under a**
sweet V-
neck
for a preppy vibe.

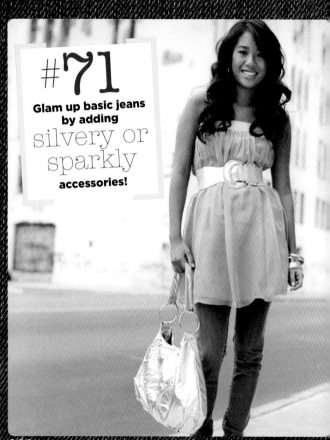

#71

**Glam up basic jeans
by adding**

silvery or
sparkly

accessories!

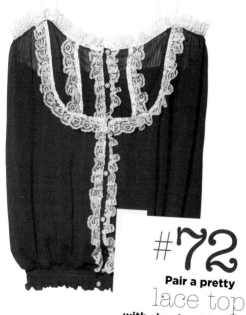

#72

Pair a pretty
lace top
**with simple white jeans for
a feminine, vintage look.**

#73

tiny flowers
look boho chic on a soft skirt.

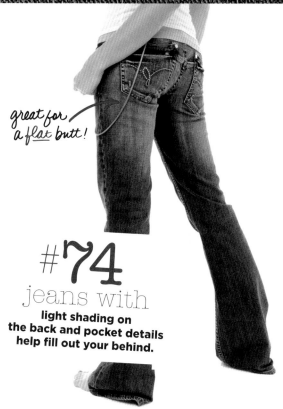

great for
a flat butt!

#74

jeans with

**light shading on
the back and pocket details
help fill out your behind.**

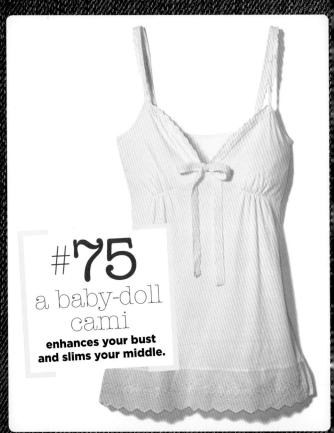

#75
a baby-doll
cami

**enhances your bust
and slims your middle.**

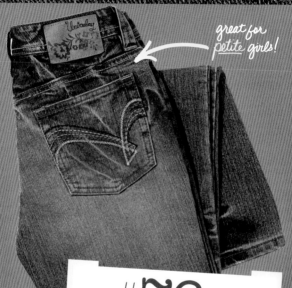

great for petite girls!

#76
high-waisted pants
make your legs look longer.

#77

balance leopard print

with solid pieces or denim, and it's perfect for class!

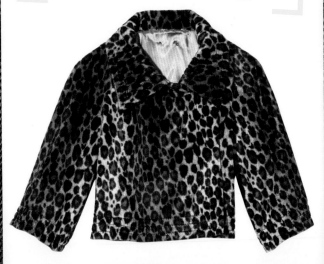

great for <u>*curvy*</u> *thighs!*

#78
bermuda shorts

with heels make your legs look miles long!

#79
slightly flared legs
look hot if you've got muscular thighs.

great for an athletic figure!

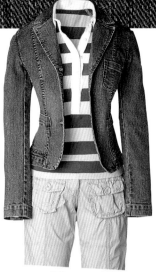

#80

a denim blazer
is versatile—you can dress it up or down.

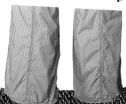

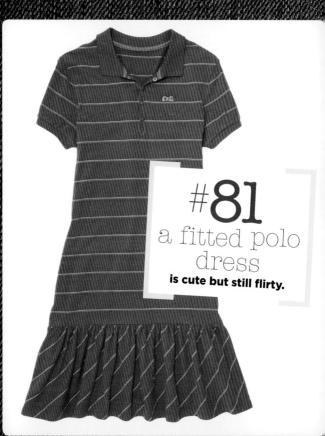

#81
a fitted polo dress
is cute but still flirty.

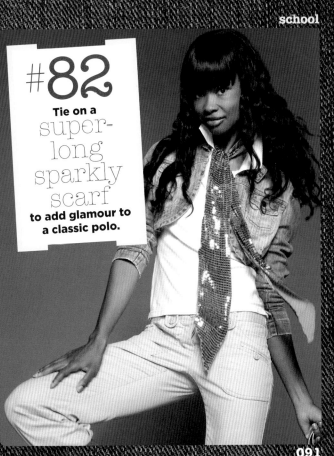

#82

Tie on a
super-
long
sparkly
scarf
**to add glamour to
a classic polo.**

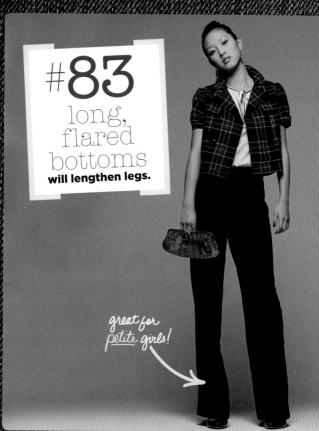

#83
long,
flared
bottoms
will lengthen legs.

great for petite girls!

#84
try a high heel
with a floral detail—it's sultry, but sweet enough for school.

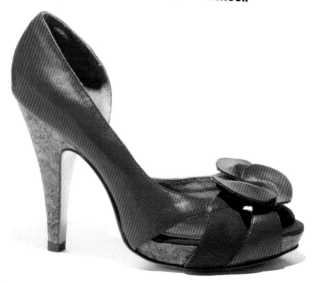

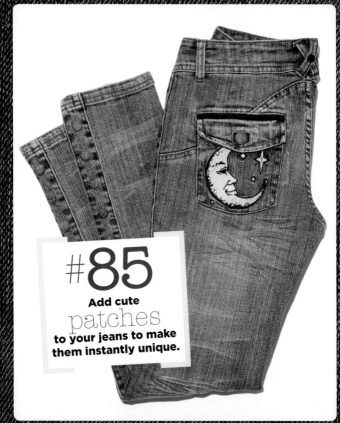

#85

Add cute
patches
to your jeans to make
them instantly unique.

#86

a bright
pair of
boots

**and a belt give
just the right fun
touch to a
neutral trench.**

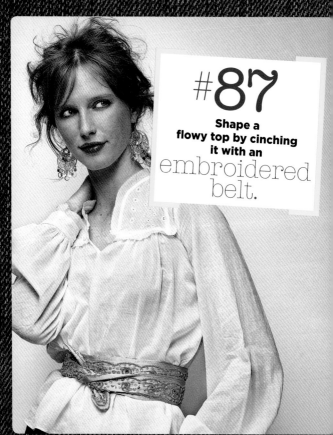

#87

Shape a flowy top by cinching it with an

embroidered belt.

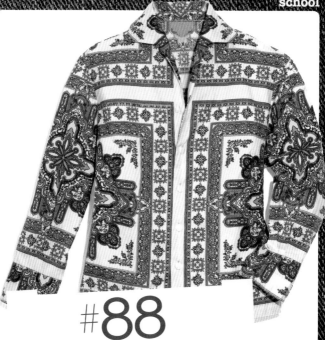

#88

a paisley-print top

**has a cool, boho vibe—
try it with a pair of cargo pants.**

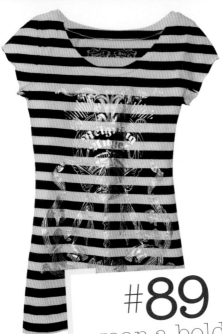

#89

wear a bold top

**with straight-leg
jeans for rocker-chic style.**

#90
add sparkly jewelry
to make a casual outfit look funkier.

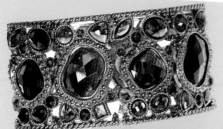

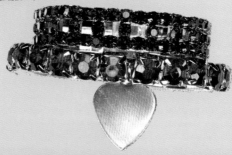

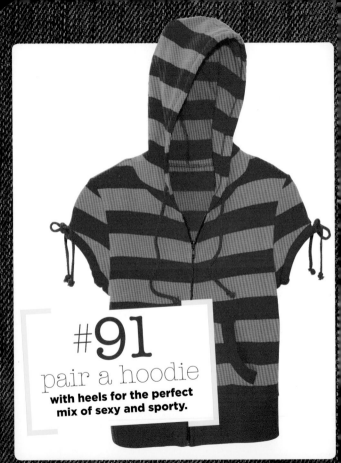

#91

pair a hoodie

with heels for the perfect mix of sexy and sporty.

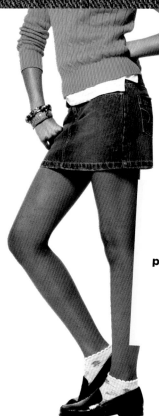

#92

Play up the preppiness of a classic cable sweater with a denim mini and cute loafers.

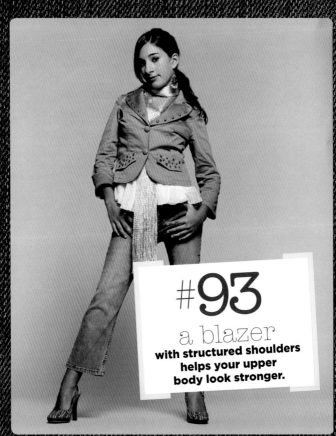

#93

a blazer
**with structured shoulders
helps your upper
body look stronger.**

#94

Mix up your
floral patterns—
**try a bold bag with a
more subtle shirt.**

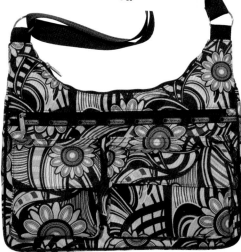

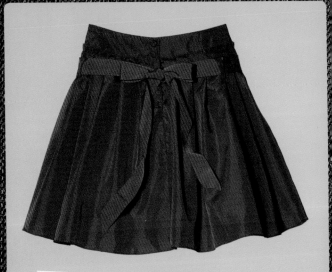

#95

a red skirt
can help you stand out in a sea of jeans.

#96

Printed

reversible belts

give you two looks in one!

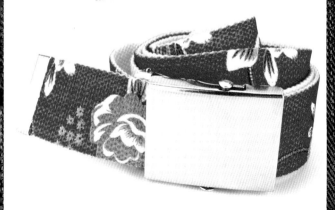

#97
wear a wrap top
to make your waist look trimmer.

make your *curves* look great!

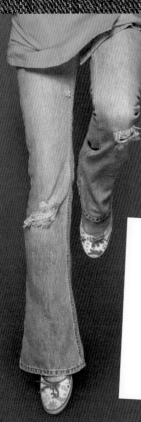

#98
girly
patterned
sneakers
**balance ripped
jeans with a touch of
femininity.**

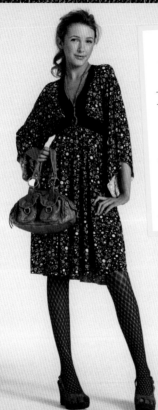

#99

mix like-colored patterns

for a unique vibe— like graphic blue patterned tights with a delicate navy floral.

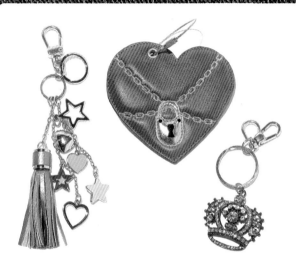

#100

Personalize your everyday book bag with

bright, fun charms.

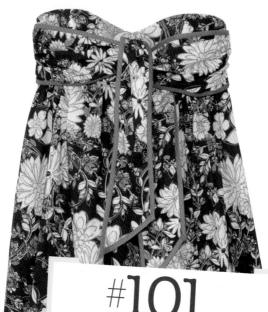

#101
a strapless top
can still be okay for school—wear a cute cardigan on top!

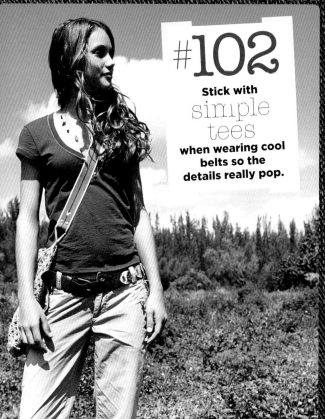

#102

Stick with
simple
tees
when wearing cool belts so the details really pop.

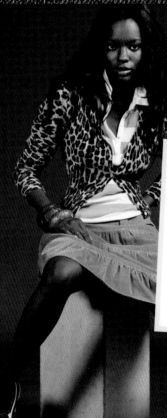

#103

When wearing

layered tops,

keep the necklines similar—but not identical—so you can see both.

#104

Collect

cute hats

**so you can save
a bad hair day!**

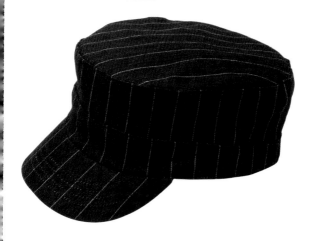

#105
long shorts
that hit just below midthigh are the right length for class.

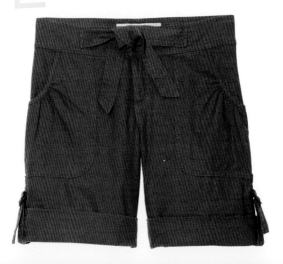

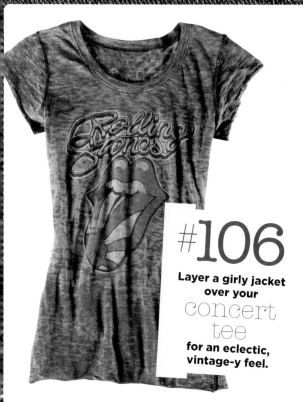

#106

Layer a girly jacket over your concert tee **for an eclectic, vintage-y feel.**

#107

Wear a
fringed scarf
over a simple floral dress for the ultimate boho effect.

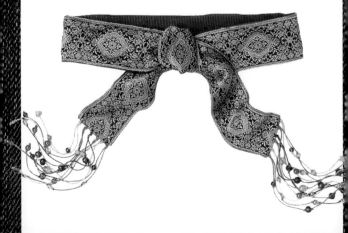

great for
a flat butt!

#108
flap pockets
add nice curves to your bottom.

#109

Pick a versatile

long
necklace—

**it can be
worn full-length or
doubled up!**

#110
patent heels
look sophisticated with a pair of skinny jeans and a black sweater.

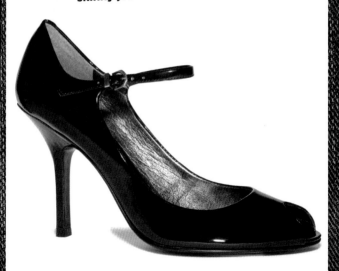

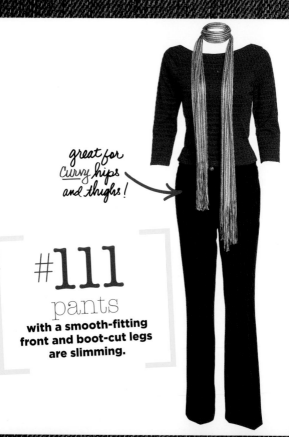

great for <u>curvy</u> hips and thighs!

#111
pants
with a smooth-fitting front and boot-cut legs are slimming.

#112

a studded belt

worn around your hips draws the eye to your cute butt!

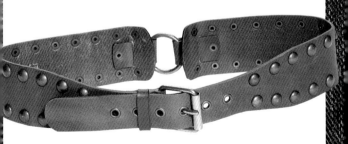

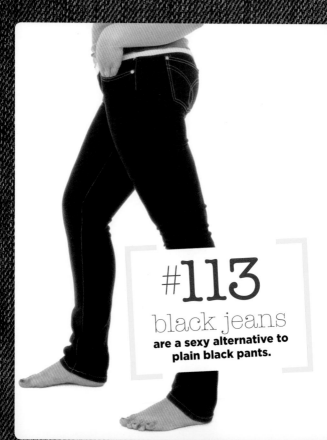

#113

black jeans

are a sexy alternative to plain black pants.

#114

wear a bangle

**high on your arm for an
unexpected yet
effortlessly cool look.**

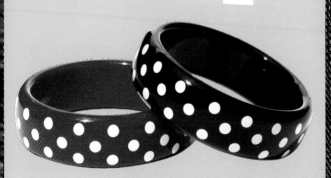

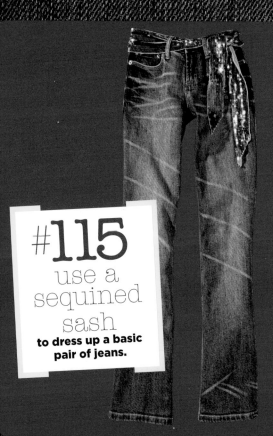

#115
use a
sequined
sash
**to dress up a basic
pair of jeans.**

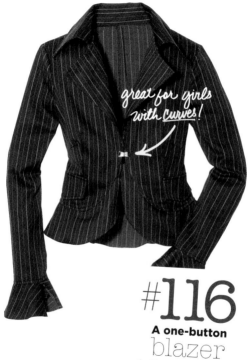

great for girls with curves!

#116

A one-button
blazer
defines your waist.

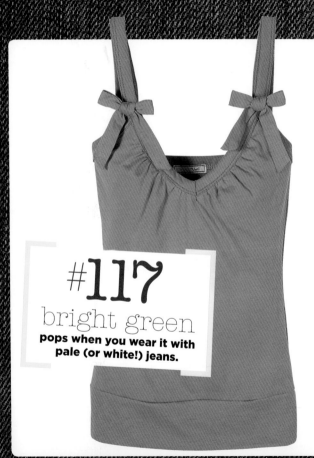

#117

bright green

pops when you wear it with pale (or white!) jeans.

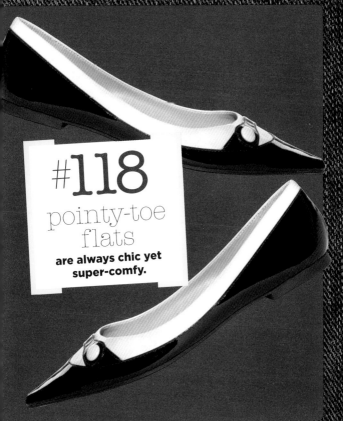

#118

pointy-toe
flats

**are always chic yet
super-comfy.**

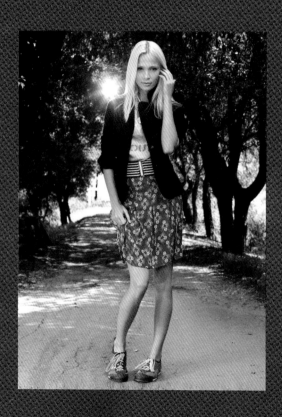

weekend

Weekends are all about comfort and relaxation—but
you can still rock your personal style, of course.
Check out this chapter for casual, hangout-friendly
outfits that'll make you feel super-cute—not sloppy!

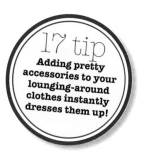

17 tip

Adding pretty
accessories to your
lounging-around
clothes instantly
dresses them up!

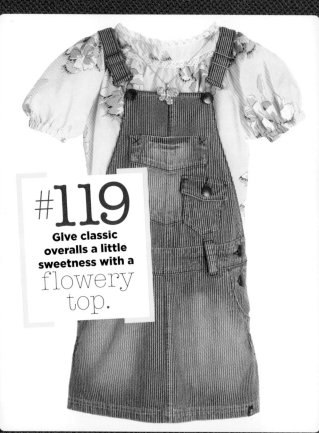

#119

Give classic overalls a little sweetness with a flowery top.

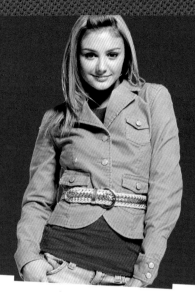

#120

Mix a
casual jacket
with a night-worthy belt—on the weekend, anything goes.

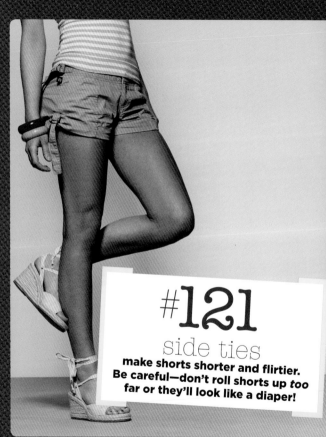

#121

side ties

**make shorts shorter and flirtier.
Be careful—don't roll shorts up *too*
far or they'll look like a diaper!**

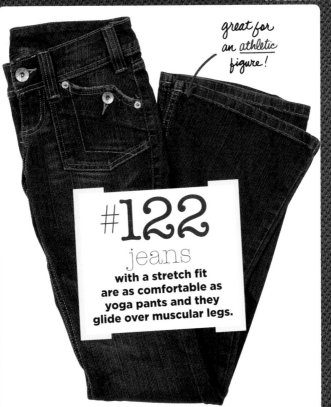

great for
an <u>athletic</u>
figure!

#122

jeans

**with a stretch fit
as are comfortable as
yoga pants and they
glide over muscular legs.**

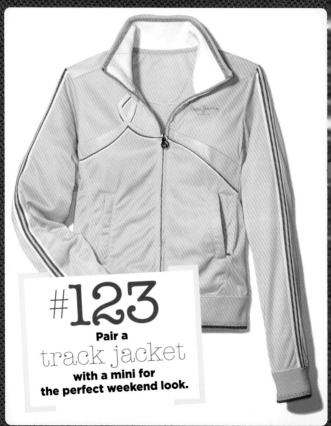

#123

Pair a
track jacket
**with a mini for
the perfect weekend look.**

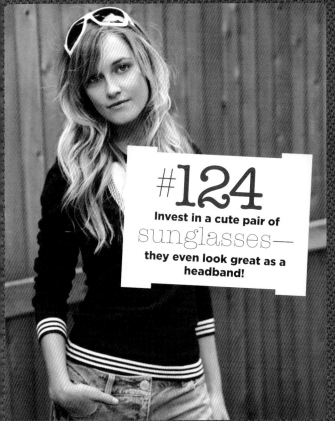

#124
Invest in a cute pair of
sunglasses—
they even look great as a
headband!

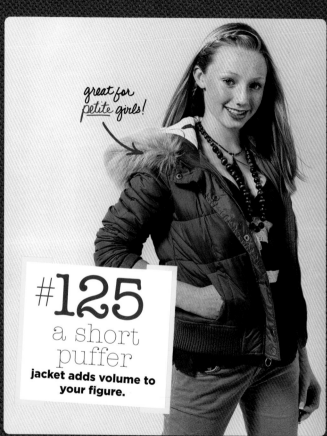

great for petite girls!

#125
a short puffer
jacket adds volume to your figure.

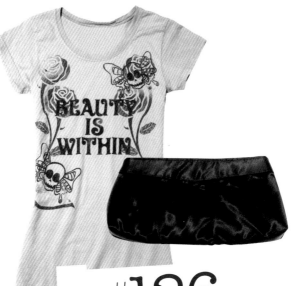

#126

You'd think a
satin purse
**would be for dresses only, but it
goes great with edgy clothes, too!**

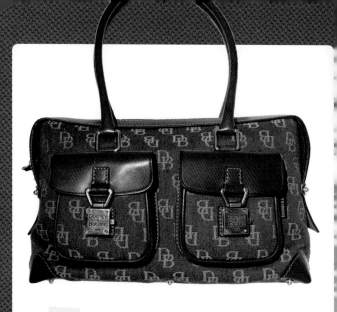

#127

A cute
designer bag
makes bargain outfits look expensive!

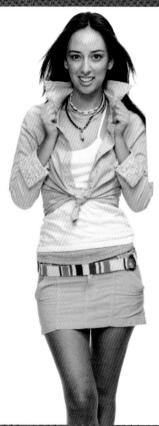

#128

When wearing a
tiny mini,
don't bare too much
on top—layering is key.

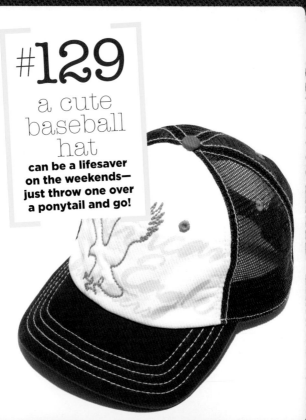

#129

a cute baseball hat

can be a lifesaver on the weekends— just throw one over a ponytail and go!

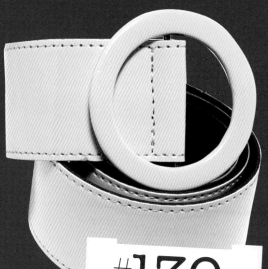

#130

Put on
a wide belt
**over a tee to cinch
your waist for a flattering
hourglass shape.**

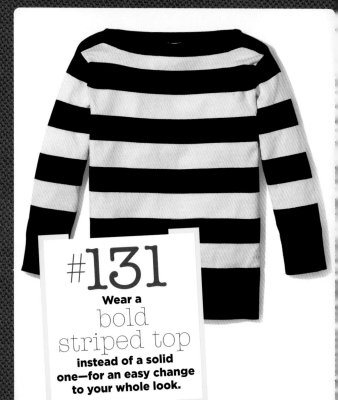

#131

Wear a
bold
striped top
**instead of a solid
one—for an easy change
to your whole look.**

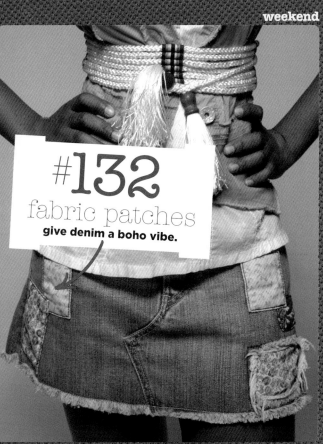

#132

fabric patches

give denim a boho vibe.

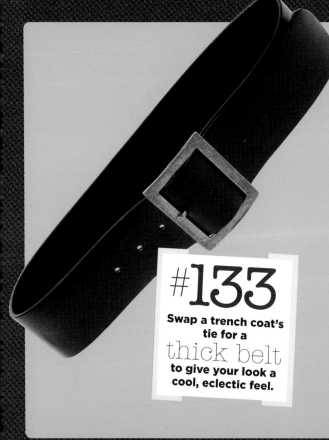

#133

Swap a trench coat's tie for a

thick belt

to give your look a cool, eclectic feel.

#134

layer your tops

**to add dimension while still
showing off your shape.**

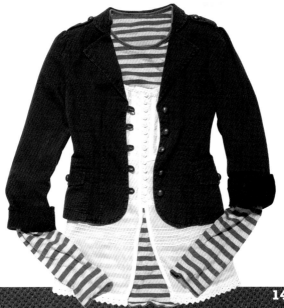

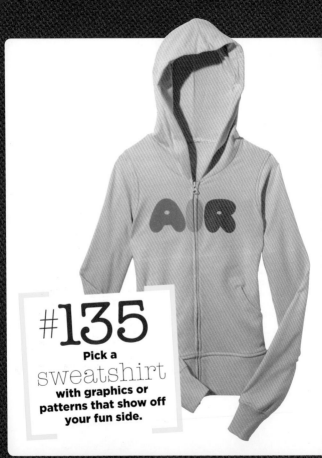

#135

Pick a
sweatshirt
**with graphics or
patterns that show off
your fun side.**

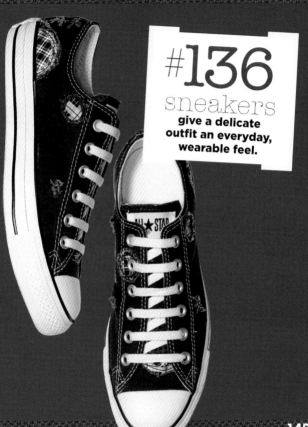

#136
sneakers
give a delicate outfit an everyday, wearable feel.

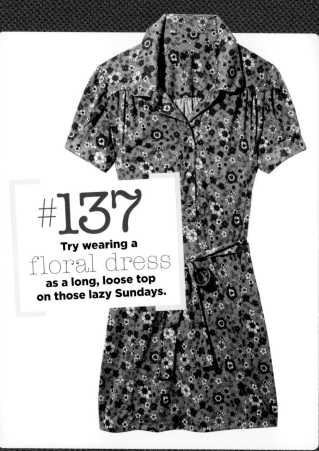

#137

Try wearing a

floral dress

**as a long, loose top
on those lazy Sundays.**

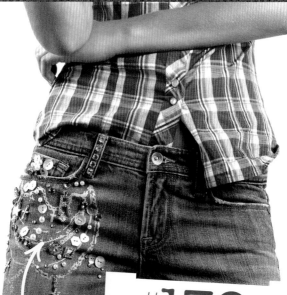

shows off
the shape
of your *hips*!

#138

For a funky edge, look for jeans with tough details like

studding.

#139
pair pretty
things,
**like a cami, with more
boyish basics, like long shorts.**

#140

Create a new-wave '80s look by wearing just *one earring.*

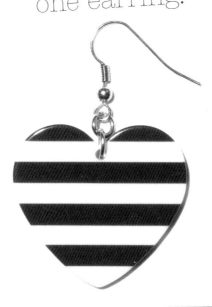

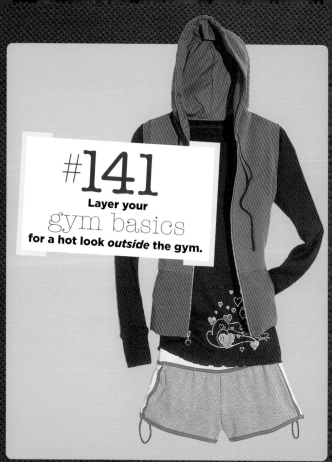

#141
Layer your
gym basics
for a hot look *outside* the gym.

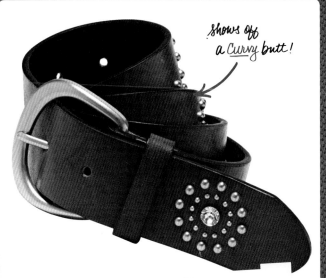

shows off a <u>curvy</u> butt!

#142

wear a rocker belt
with low-rise jeans to highlight your bottom.

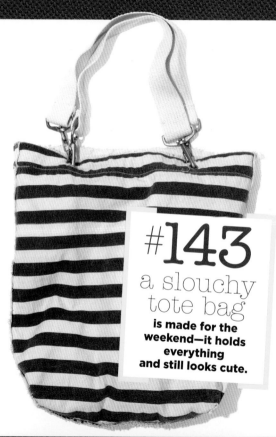

#143

a slouchy tote bag

is made for the weekend—it holds everything and still looks cute.

#144
a funky hat
is the perfect way to hide that messy weekend hair!

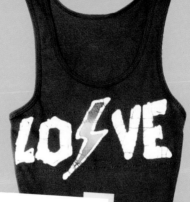

#145

Pair a
rock tee
**with tough accessories
like a studded bracelet
or a cool wallet
chain for an edgy look.**

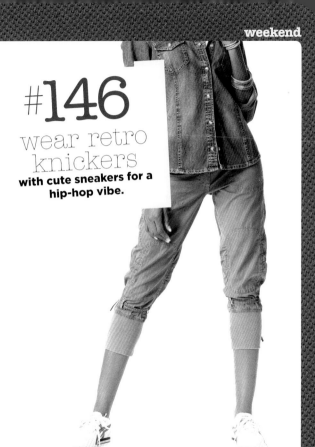

#146

wear retro knickers

with cute sneakers for a hip-hop vibe.

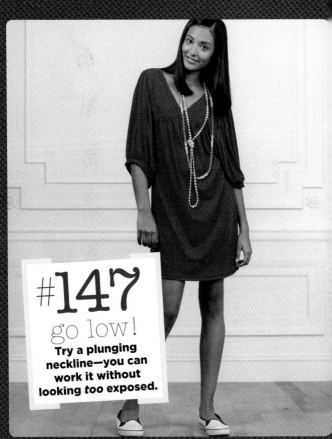

#147
go low!
Try a plunging neckline—you can work it without looking *too* exposed.

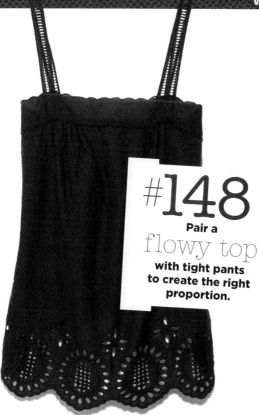

#148
Pair a
flowy top
**with tight pants
to create the right
proportion.**

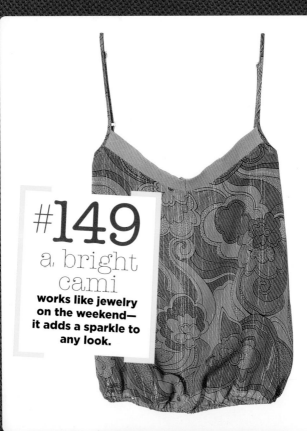

#149

a bright cami

**works like jewelry
on the weekend—
it adds a sparkle to
any look.**

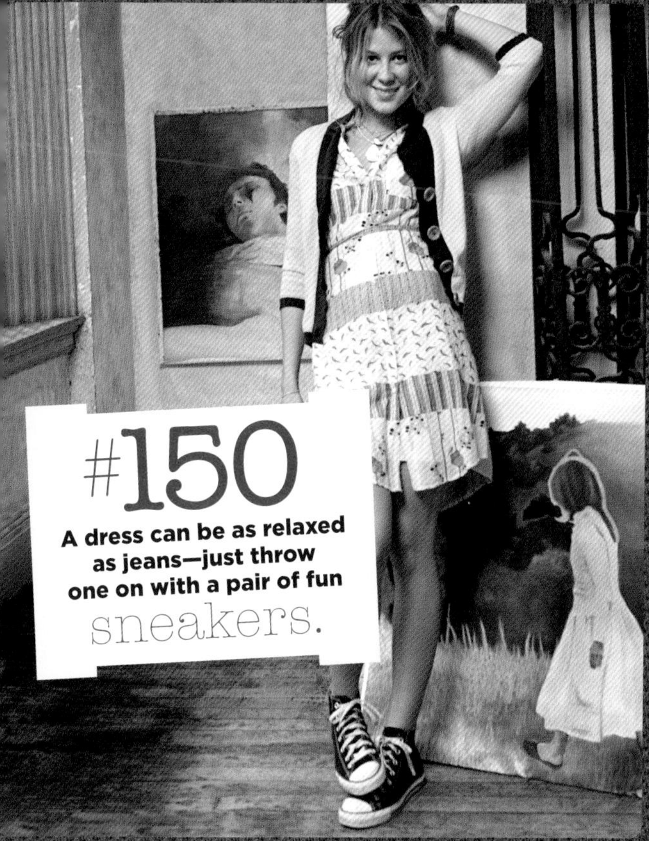

#150

**A dress can be as relaxed
as jeans—just throw
one on with a pair of fun**
sneakers.

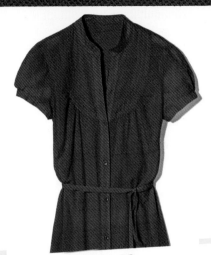

#151
Unbutton the bottom of a
button-up dress
over jeans so it's comfier and even cuter.

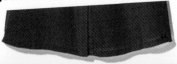

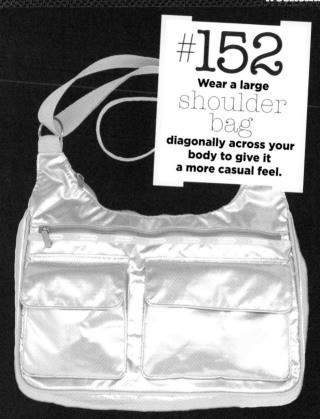

#152

Wear a large
shoulder
bag
diagonally across your body to give it a more casual feel.

#153

Give a solid tee more of an earthgirl feel by throwing on an oversize

wooden necklace.

#154

a funky flat

**is a comfy yet stylish
alternative to sneakers.**

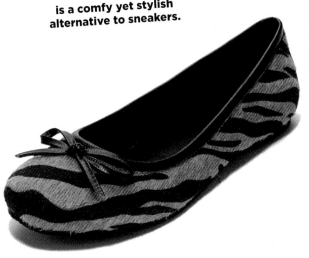

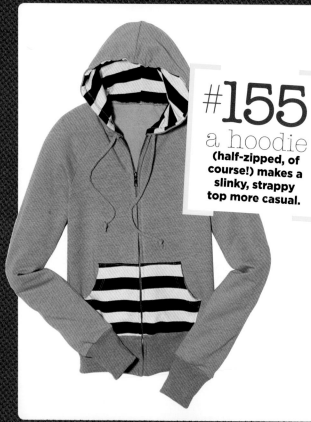

#155

a hoodie
(half-zipped, of course!) makes a slinky, strappy top more casual.

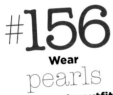

#156
Wear
pearls
with a sporty outfit to add a feminine touch.

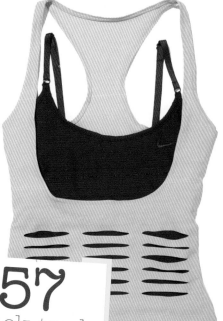

#157
a Y-back tank
**shows off your back
in a flirty yet sporty way.**

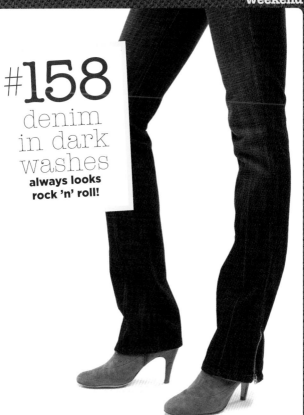

#158
denim
in dark
washes
**always looks
rock 'n' roll!**

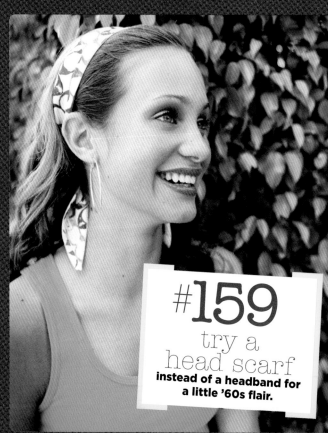

#159

try a
head scarf

**instead of a headband for
a little '60s flair.**

#160
a double-breasted
jacket adds curves to your shape.

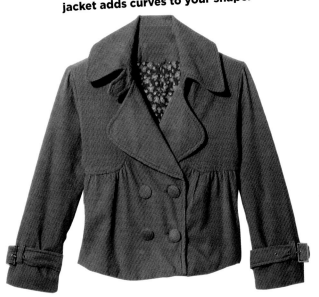

#161

cargos

are great for hanging out: wear 'em loose, roll 'em up, and you're ready to go.

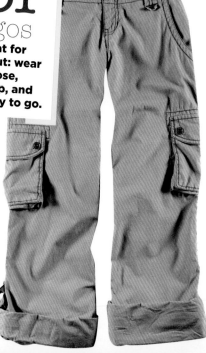

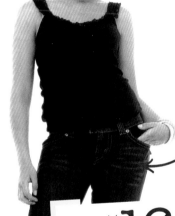

great for a pear shape!

#162
jeans with slanted pockets
make hips appear narrower.

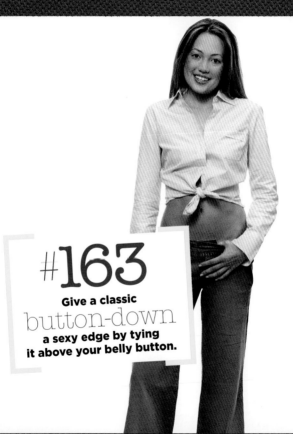

#163

Give a classic
button-down
a sexy edge by tying
it above your belly button.

#164

**If you love
your long legs,**
short
shorts
**will let you put them
front and center.**

*great for
tall girls!*

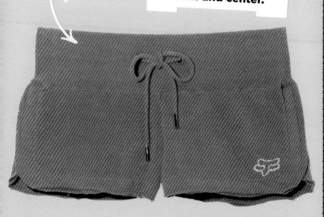

#165
wedge boots
are more comfy than they look—the sole gives you height but doesn't hurt like heels can.

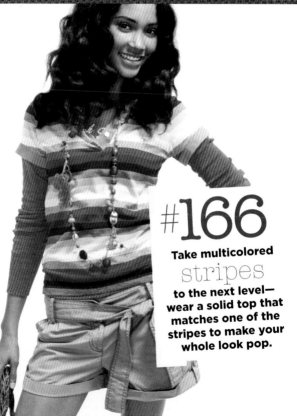

#166

Take multicolored
stripes
**to the next level—
wear a solid top that
matches one of the
stripes to make your
whole look pop.**

#167
a peasant skirt

**and a slouchy bag
give you a boho look.**

#168
classic kicks
**look as cute with
jeans as they do with a mini!**

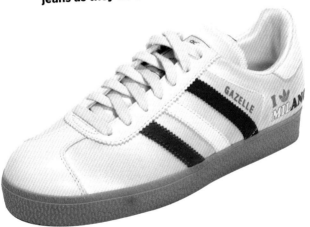

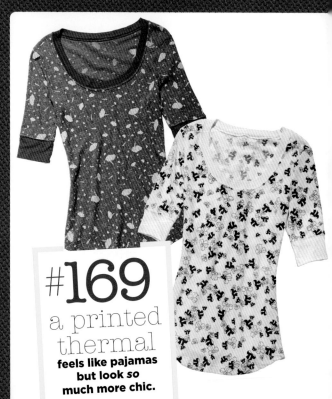

#169

a printed thermal

**feels like pajamas
but look *so*
much more chic.**

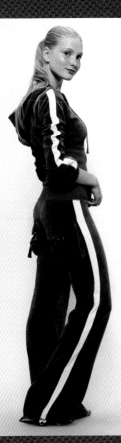

#170

velour

gives sweatpants an old-school hip-hop vibe.

great for an hourglass shape!

#171
a snug-fitting tee
adds definition to your upper body.

#172
wooden platforms
have a casual look but are comfy enough for the mall.

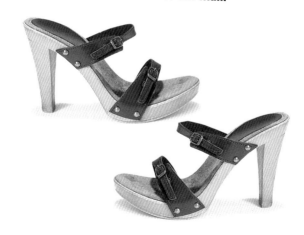

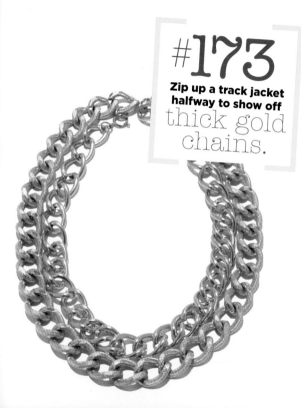

#173

Zip up a track jacket halfway to show off thick gold chains.

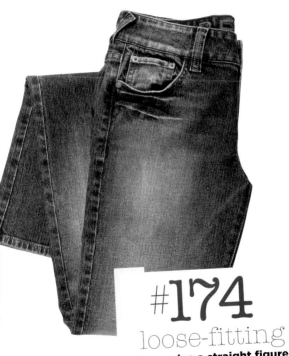

#174
loose-fitting
**jeans give a straight figure
a curvier look.**

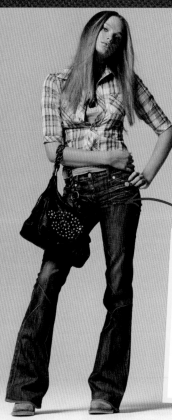

great for curry hips!

#175

Pants with slant pockets **in the front add interest but don't add bulk.**

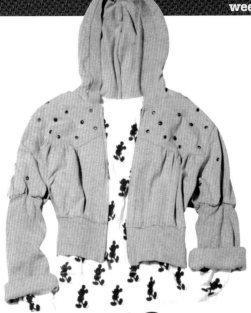

#176

a gray cropped hoodie
looks great with almost *any* color palette.

#177

A worn-in tee and a cropped leather jacket **were practically made for each other.**

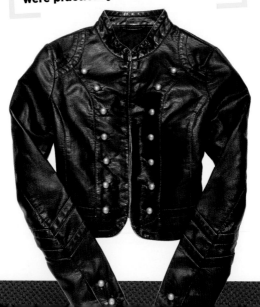

#178
overalls
**are a comfy staple—try
some in a bright color!**

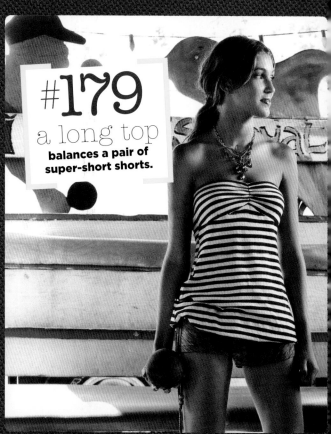

#179
a long top
balances a pair of super-short shorts.

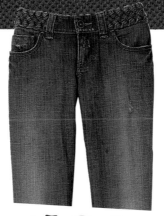

#180
stretchy low-rise
jeans flatter curves in a sexy way.

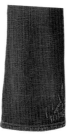

#181

Express yourself with *charms* **that make a statement!**

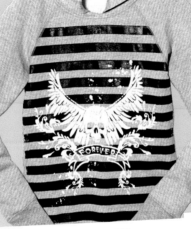

#182
a hoodie
tied around your waist makes a cute belt *and* shows off your shape!

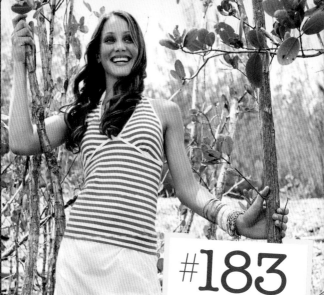

#183
turn a
dress into
a skirt
**by layering a tank
top over it!**

#184
pair slingbacks

**in a pretty floral pattern with a sundress
for an ultra-feminine yet comfy outfit.**

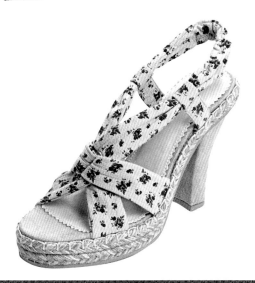

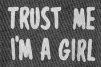

#185

Find a tee that hits
below the
hips—
**it will look cute
peeking out from
under a hoodie.**

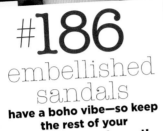

#186
embellished sandals
have a boho vibe—so keep the rest of your look simple and sweet!

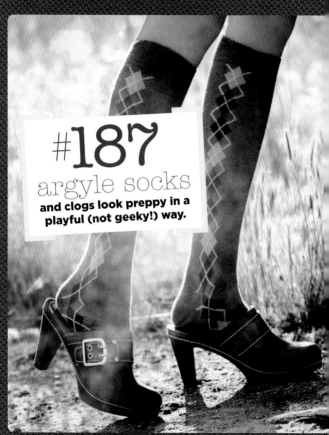

#187

argyle socks

and clogs look preppy in a playful (not geeky!) way.

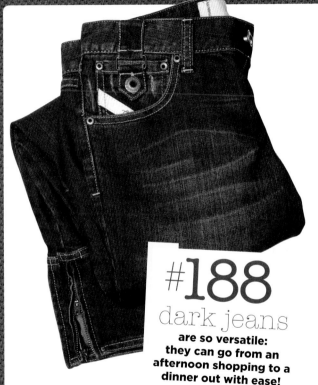

#188
dark jeans
**are so versatile:
they can go from an
afternoon shopping to a
dinner out with ease!**

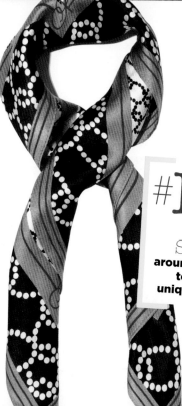

#189

Wrap a scarf **around your wrist to make a unique bracelet.**

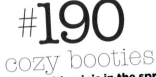

#190
cozy booties
look cute with minis in the spring and fall. They'll still look good with jeans in the winter.

#191

Put a long cardigan over short shorts **to play down their length.**

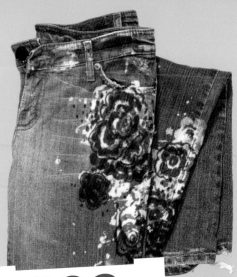

#192
bleach spots
give denim an edgy feel.

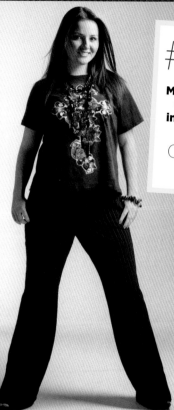

#193

Mix a vintage-y tee with menswear-inspired pants and sneakers for a

cool-girl effect.

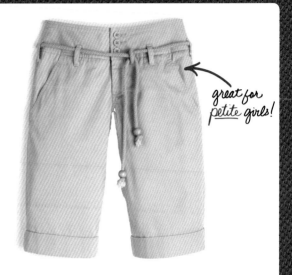

great for <u>petite</u> girls!

#194
midthigh-length
shorts elongate your figure by showing just the right amount of leg.

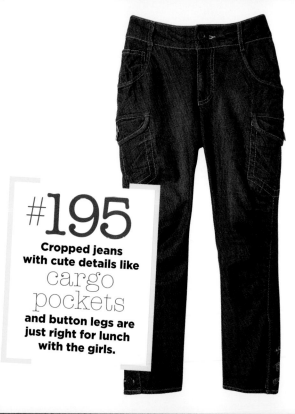

#195

Cropped jeans with cute details like cargo pockets **and button legs are just right for lunch with the girls.**

#196
a fun
necklace
**gives a relaxed
outfit a fun twist.**

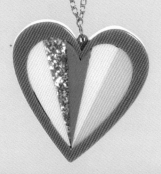

#197

Rewhiten

sneaker soles

with whitewall car tire cleanser.

#198

a flowy
dress

**is a dream on a hot
day—the natural
movement of the
fabric keeps you cool.**

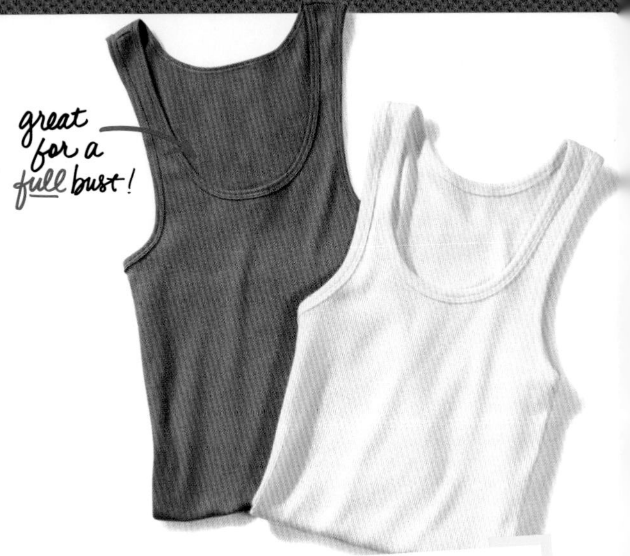

great
for a
full bust!

#199

wear two
contrasting tanks
to hide bra straps.

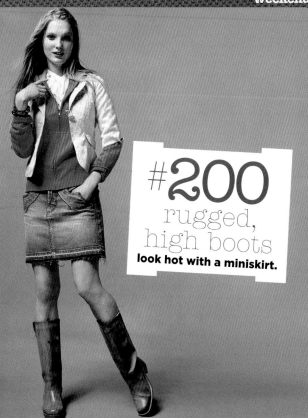

#200
rugged,
high boots
look hot with a miniskirt.

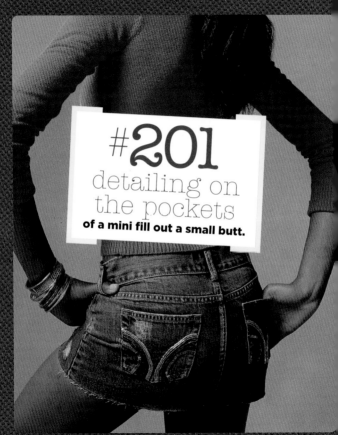

#201

detailing on
the pockets
of a mini fill out a small butt.

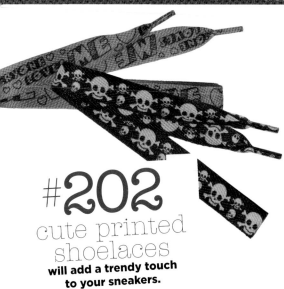

#202
cute printed
shoelaces
**will add a trendy touch
to your sneakers.**

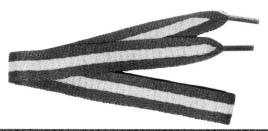

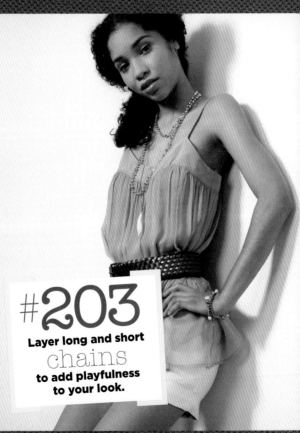

#203
Layer long and short *chains* to add playfulness to your look.

#204

Pants with a

feminine
detail

**look fresh with printed
sneakers.**

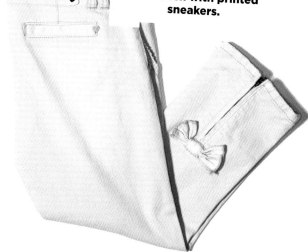

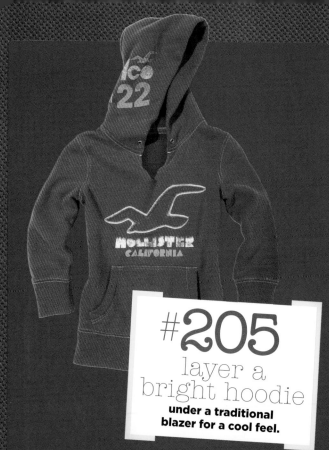

#205
layer a bright hoodie
under a traditional blazer for a cool feel.

#206

Pair a denim mini with navy
sailor-striped wedges
for a classic preppy look.

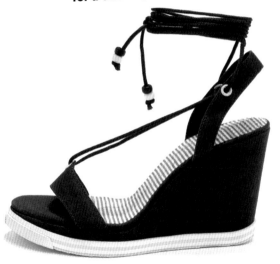

#207

a romper

**in a soft cotton material
is as comfy as sweats!**

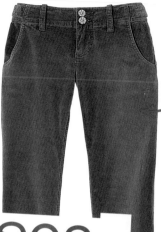

great for petite girls!

#208

Pants with a
hip-hugging
fit elongate a short torso.

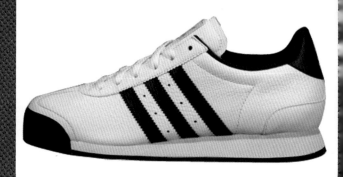

#209

Just because you don't play soccer doesn't mean you can't make any outfit a bit more sporty with

soccer sneakers.

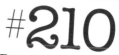

#210

**Transform your jeans—
cuff them to make instant**
capris!

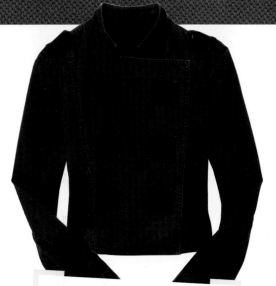

#211
put a
cropped jacket
**over a white T-shirt
to spruce up a plain outfit.**

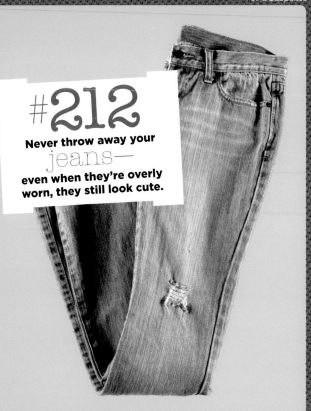

#212

Never throw away your
jeans—
**even when they're overly
worn, they still look cute.**

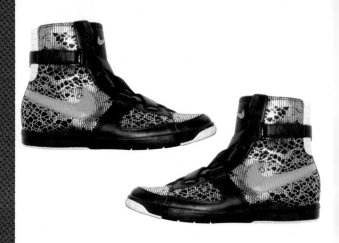

#213

Finish your outfit in an unexpected way: go for sneakers with bold laces or a

funky design.

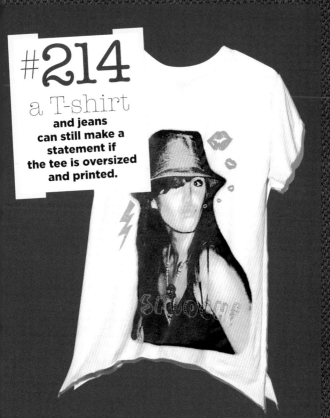

#214

a T-shirt

**and jeans
can still make a
statement if
the tee is oversized
and printed.**

#215

Add a splash of color to an understated all-white outfit by layering a bright yellow tank **underneath.**

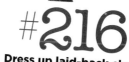

#216

**Dress up laid-back clothes
with a shiny bag in a**
bold color.

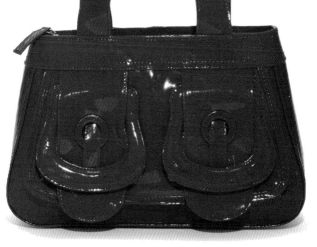

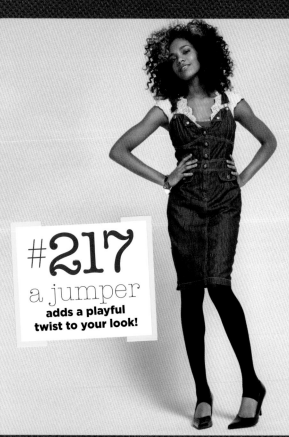

#217

a jumper
**adds a playful
twist to your look!**

#218

Slip on a pair of relaxed

old-school
sneakers—

**they add more personality
than gym sneakers.**

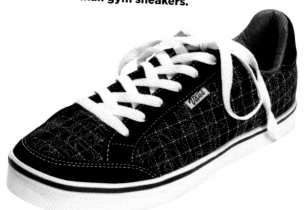

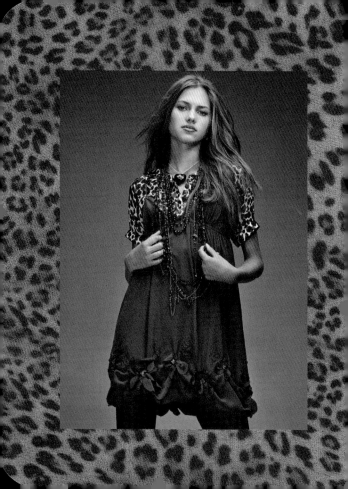

party

Round up your girls and hit the town...or even just your friend's house! Parties are the perfect opportunities to experiment with your style. This chapter is full of glam, eye-catching ideas.

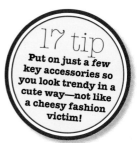

17 tip
Put on just a few key accessories so you look trendy in a cute way—not like a cheesy fashion victim!

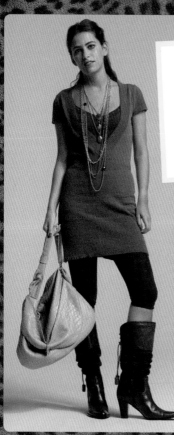

#219

slouchy
boots
**make any look cooler
and more casual.**

#220
gold or silver sandals
look totally hot with a bold dress.

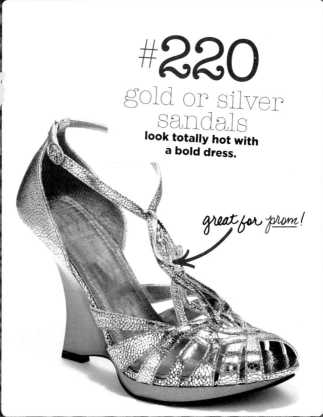

great for prom!

great for _petite girls!_

#221

dresses

that are short and flouncy won't overpower a small frame.

#222

Put on brightly colored

plastic jewelry

**with going-out clothes
to give your outfit a sweet feel.**

#223
leopard
accessories
**are timeless—all you need is one
little touch to make an impact!**

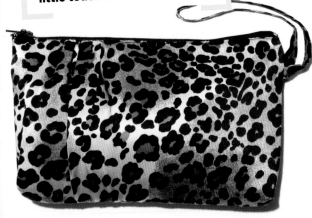

great for *prom*!

#224
a wide satin waistband
fakes an hourglass shape.

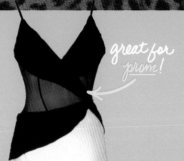

great for prom!

#225

Try a dress with
semisheer panels
**at the waist to reveal nice
abs in an understated way.**

#226

Tone down a fancy dress by pairing it with a

sporty
hoodie.

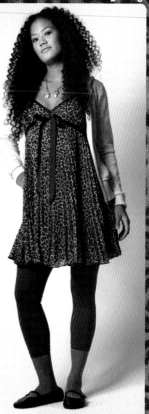

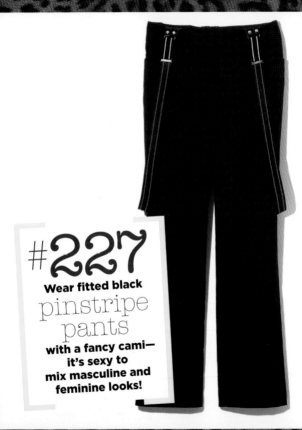

#227

Wear fitted black

pinstripe
pants

**with a fancy cami—
it's sexy to
mix masculine and
feminine looks!**

#228
kick
pleats
**show off long legs
in a playful way.**

*great for
<u>tall</u> girls!*

#229
a flutter-sleeved top
delicately frames strong arms.

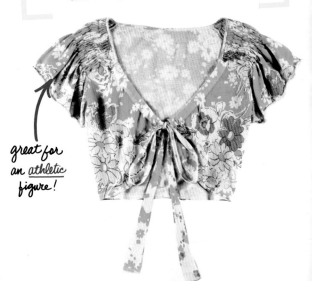

great for an athletic figure!

great for prom!

#230

Wear a feminine dress with sparkly accents **and you won't have to spend any money on jewelry!**

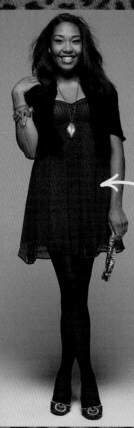

#231

Choose a dress with a *high waist* **to conceal a curvy tummy.**

great for a curvy middle!

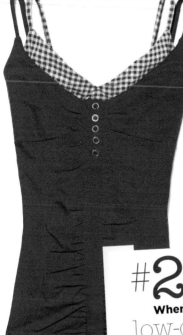

#232

When wearing a
low-cut top,
layer another tank underneath it so you don't show *too* much.

#233

When you wear high heels, bring jeweled or beaded flip flops **so you can switch your shoes if your feet start to hurt.**

great for prom!

#234
wear a skinny belt

**over a top to show off a
slim waist and curvy hips.**

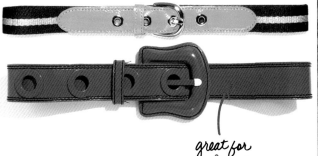

*great for
an hourglass
shape!*

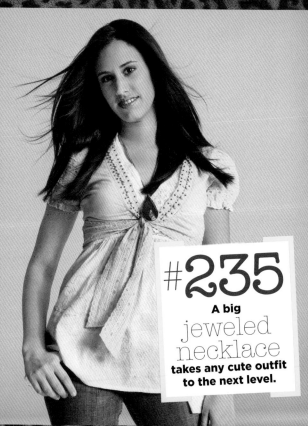

#235

A big
jeweled
necklace
**takes any cute outfit
to the next level.**

#236

A dress with an

asymmetrical hem

reveals just a flash of leg: it's more elegant than a mini.

great for prom!

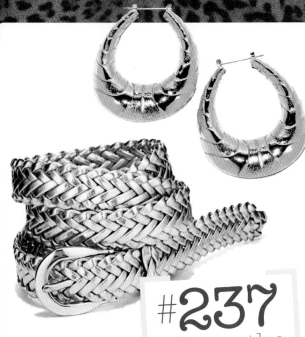

#237

pile on the bling!

Wear metallic hoops to accent a gold belt.

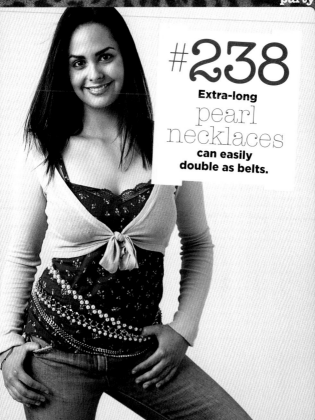

#238

Extra-long
pearl
necklaces
**can easily
double as belts.**

great for an athletic figure!

#239

a high neck halter top

accentuates shoulders in the most flattering way.

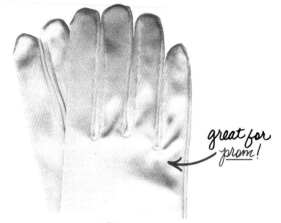

great for prom!

#240

remove gloves

at dinner, but wear them on the dance floor!

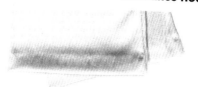

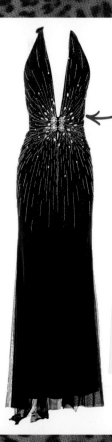

great for <u>prom</u>!

#241

Keep a

low-cut dress

in place by securing the fabric to your skin with double-sided tape.

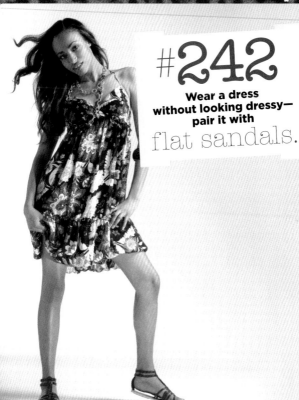

#242

**Wear a dress
without looking dressy—
pair it with**

flat sandals.

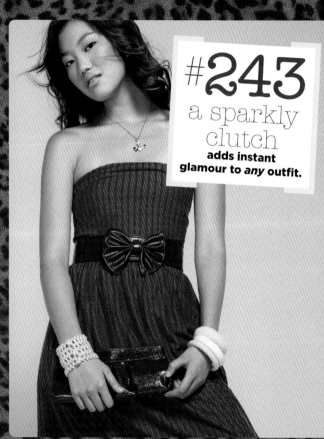

#243

a sparkly clutch **adds instant glamour to *any* outfit.**

#244

Make a little black dress cuter by layering it

over jeans.

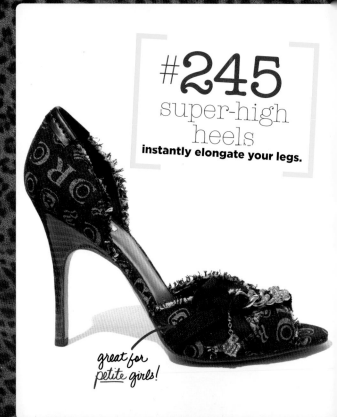

#245
super-high
heels
instantly elongate your legs.

great for petite girls!

#246
use bright
accessories
**to add color to a
neutral-toned outfit.**

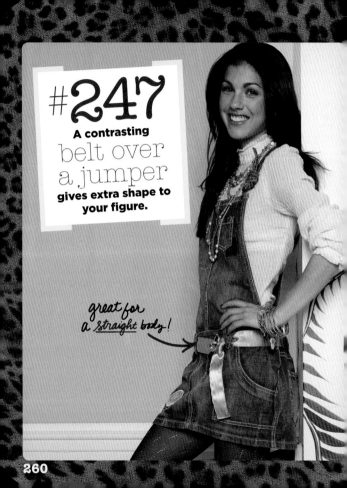

#247

A contrasting
belt over
a jumper
**gives extra shape to
your figure.**

*great for
a straight body!*

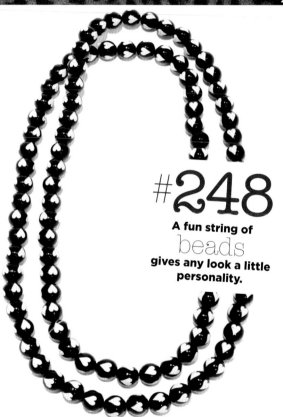

#248

A fun string of
beads
**gives any look a little
personality.**

#249

oxfords

are good for school—but Oxfords with a heel are great for a night out!

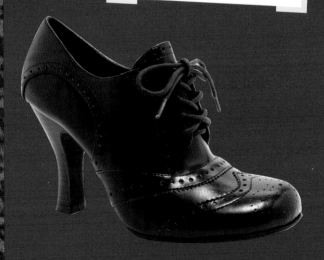

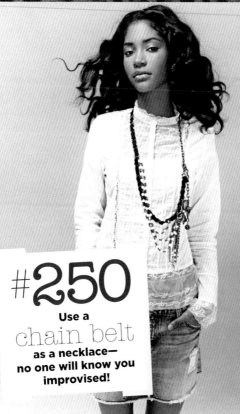

#250

Use a
chain belt
**as a necklace—
no one will know you
improvised!**

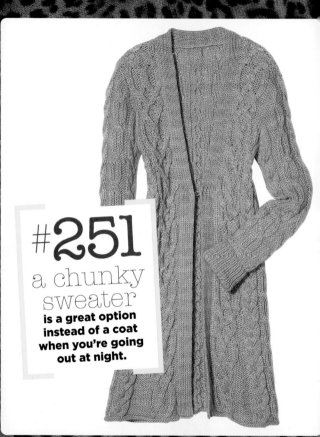

#251

a chunky sweater

**is a great option
instead of a coat
when you're going
out at night.**

#252

Accessorize with just a
pile of bangles
**and a men's watch for
the ultimate cool statement.**

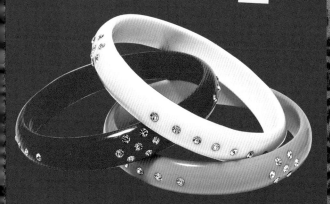

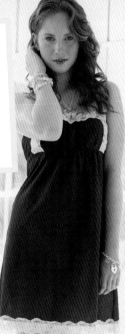

#253

Pick a
girly dress
**with lace trim.
It's sexy like lingerie—
but less revealing!**

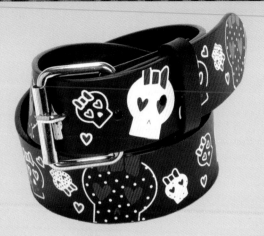

#254
an edgy belt
can update an otherwise boring outfit.

#255

Fasten

ankle-strap shoes

over jeans for an eclectic touch.

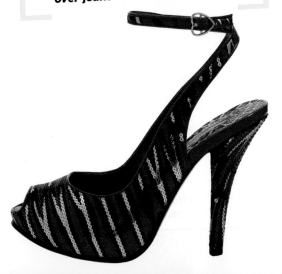

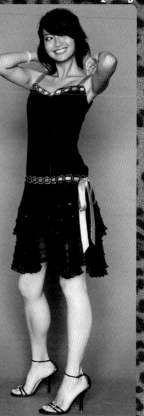

#256
Try a skirt with
ruffled
tiers
or layered chiffon to
create curves.

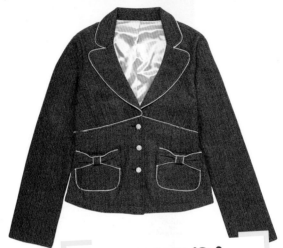

#257

Balance a tiny mini with a

boxy jacket—

it's fun to play with cool shapes.

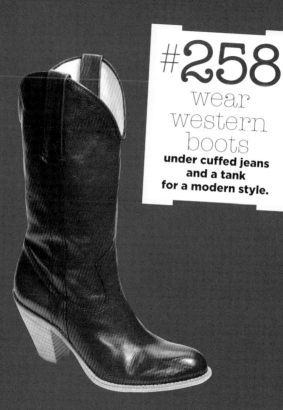

#258

wear western boots

under cuffed jeans and a tank for a modern style.

#259

For a dress with heavy beading or detailing on the bodice, add a

sparkly bracelet

to draw the eye to the rest of your body, too!

great for prom!

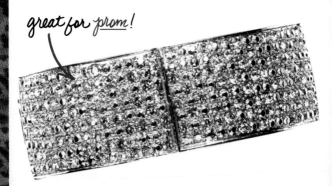

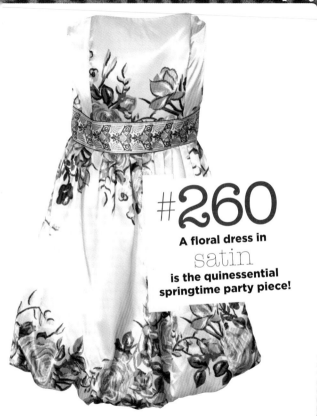

#260

A floral dress in

satin

**is the quinessential
springtime party piece!**

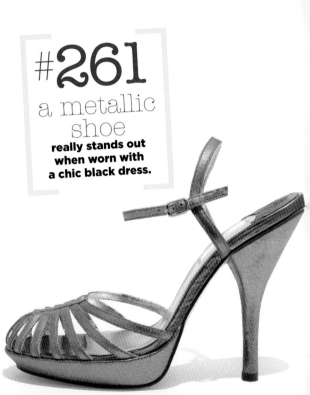

#261
a metallic shoe
really stands out when worn with a chic black dress.

#262

an extra-long
pendant necklace

is a pretty centerpiece for any look.

great for a curvy frame!

#263
an A-line dress
creates a sleek-looking silhouette.

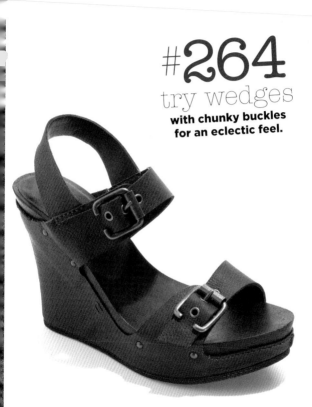

#264
try wedges
**with chunky buckles
for an eclectic feel.**

#265

Layer a rocker

vest over a minidress

for an edgy (yet classy!) look.

#266

Transform a simple dress by putting a low-slung

leather belt

over it.

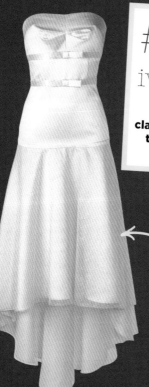

#267

ivory satin

isn't just for weddings—it's a classic choice for prom that looks great on *any* skin tone.

great for a slim middle!

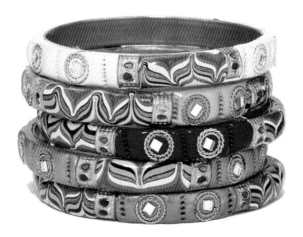

#268
put bangles
***over* your sleeve to give your
outfit a totally
sophisticated vibe.**

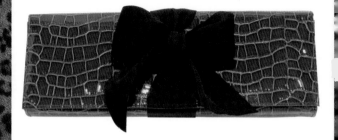

#269
a little clutch
**in a crazy bold color can work
with almost *any* dress.**

#270

double up

**your legwear—
colored tights under
fishnets look foxy
and keep you warm.**

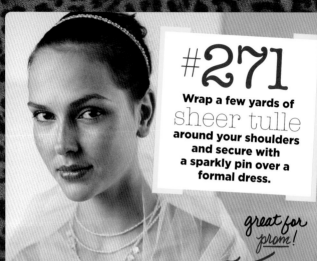

#271

Wrap a few yards of sheer tulle **around your shoulders and secure with a sparkly pin over a formal dress.**

great for prom!

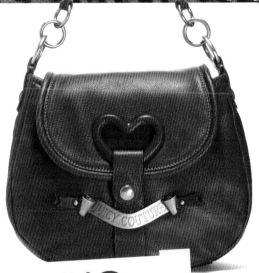

#272

Don't bring a

giant bag

to a party! Make sure you carry a bag that is *just* big enough for essentials!

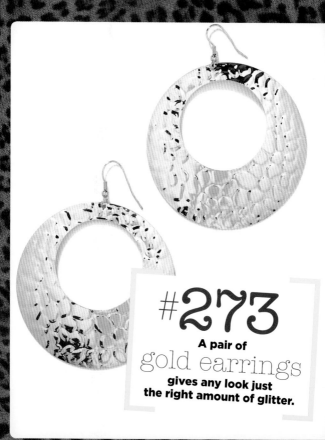

#273

A pair of
gold earrings
**gives any look just
the right amount of glitter.**

#274

a corset belt

worn over loose layers will give you a sexy shape.

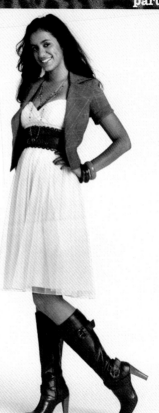

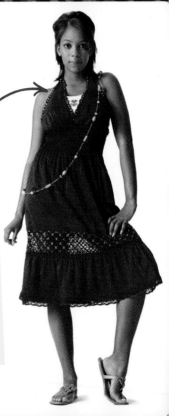

great for a full bust!

#275

When you wear
**a halter
dress**
try a strapless or
a halter bra so your
straps don't show.

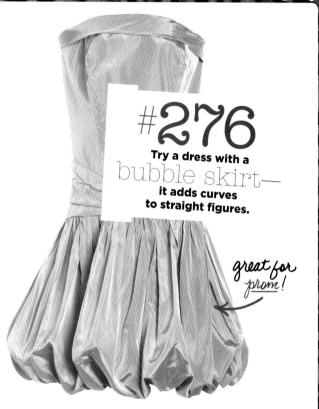

#276

Try a dress with a
bubble skirt—
**it adds curves
to straight figures.**

great for prom!

#277

a metallic bag

**is so versatile—
it goes with any dress color!**

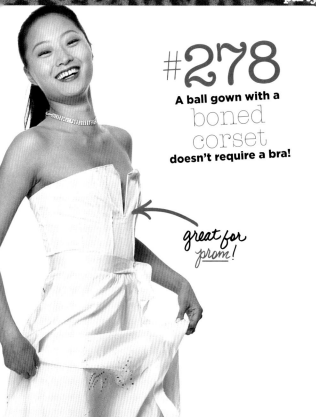

#278

A ball gown with a
boned
corset
doesn't require a bra!

*great for
prom!*

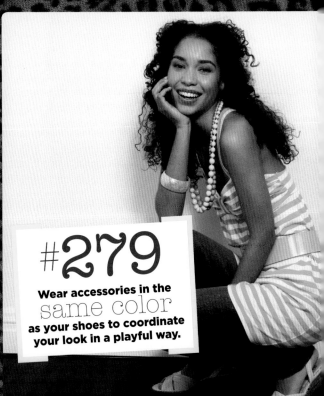

#279

Wear accessories in the same color **as your shoes to coordinate your look in a playful way.**

great for __prom__!

#280

When attending a very formal event, choose a dress in

satin or silk—

the most elegant fabrics.

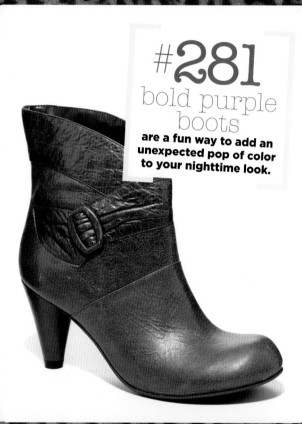

#281
bold purple boots
are a fun way to add an unexpected pop of color to your nighttime look.

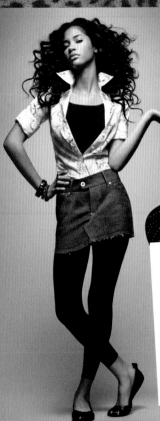

#282

Try a mini with
footless
tights
**for a little more
coverage.**

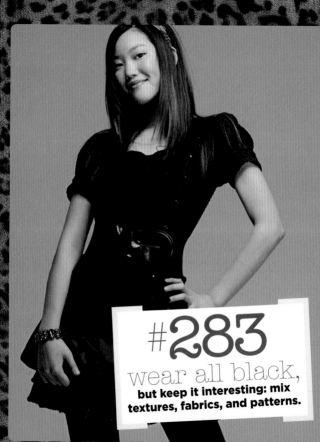

#283

wear all black,
**but keep it interesting: mix
textures, fabrics, and patterns.**

#284

A dress with a full,

flouncy hem

makes hips look slimmer in contrast.

great for <u>curvy</u> hips!

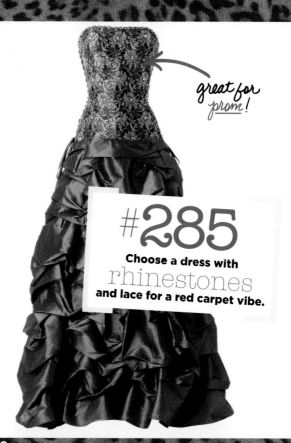

great for *prom!*

#285

Choose a dress with
rhinestones
and lace for a red carpet vibe.

#286

Put a multistrand

necklace

on—or mix at
least three necklaces
yourself.

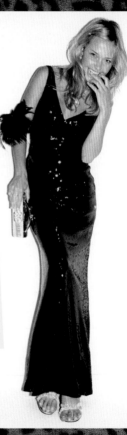

great for *prom!*

#287

**Stand out
with a dress that has**
feather
details—
it's fun and flashy!

#288

**Trade up your jeans from
basic styles:**

sweet details
will make your look unique.

#289
wear a big-buckle belt
to draw the eye to your hips.

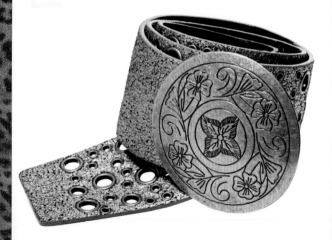

great for a <u>curvy</u> middle!

#290

an empire-waist

cut glides over your tummy.

#291

Add a touch of glitz with a
spangled bag.

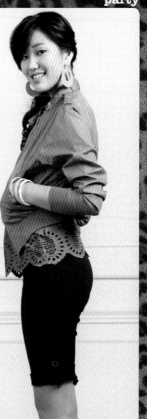

#292
a boxy jacket
is the right proportion—and looks cute—with fitted long shorts.

#293

A shoe with a pointy toe and 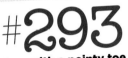 **high heel makes legs look long and lean.**

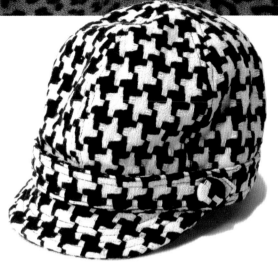

#294

a bold cap

**can stand alone—no need to wear
earrings or a necklace with it.**

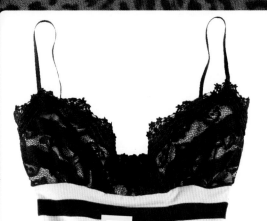

#295
black and
white stripes
make you stand out in *any* room.

#296

A skirt or dress with a
floaty
hem
**will make boyish legs
look curvier.**

*great for
a straight body!*

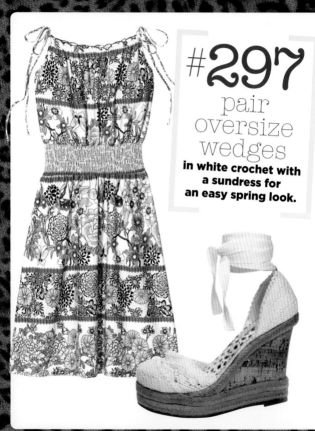

#297

pair
oversize
wedges

**in white crochet with
a sundress for
an easy spring look.**

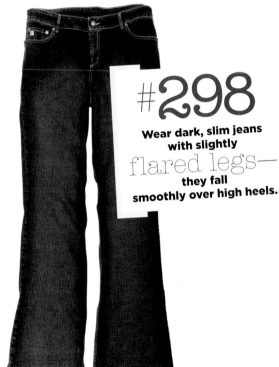

#298

Wear dark, slim jeans with slightly flared legs— **they fall smoothly over high heels.**

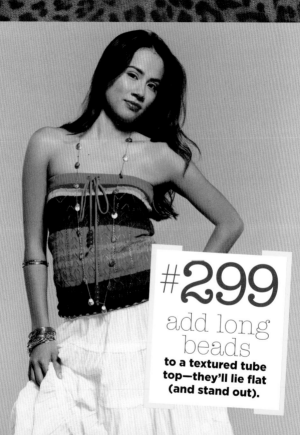

#299

add long beads

to a textured tube top—they'll lie flat (and stand out).

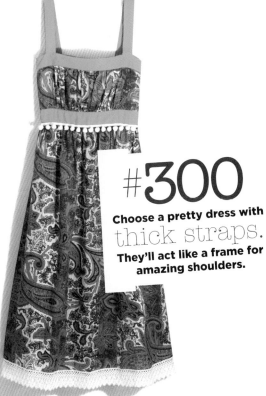

#300

Choose a pretty dress with thick straps. **They'll act like a frame for amazing shoulders.**

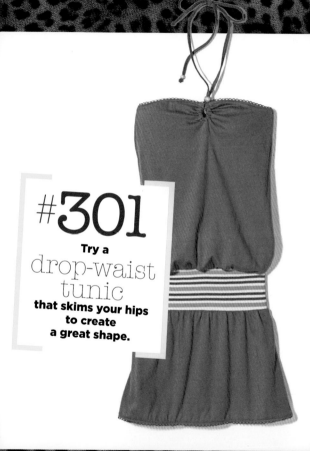

#301

Try a
drop-waist
tunic
**that skims your hips
to create
a great shape.**

#302

one big piece

of jewelry can make a stronger impact than a lot of little pieces.

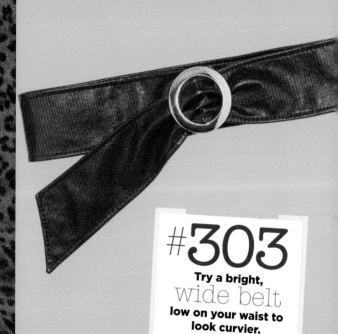

#303

Try a bright,
wide belt
**low on your waist to
look curvier.**

#304

There's really only one occasion where you can wear long gloves— **so take full advantage of the classic glamour of satin—from fingertips to elbow!**

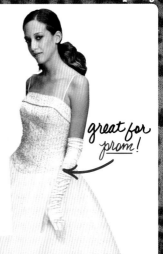

great for prom!

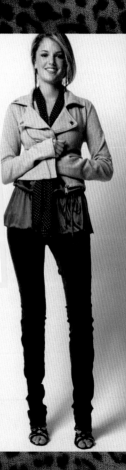

#305

low-slung,
skinny
**jeans always fit a straight
figure perfectly.**

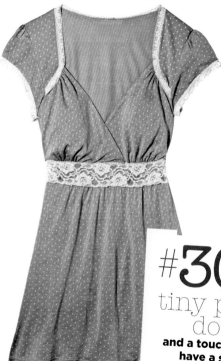

#306
tiny polka dots
and a touch of lace have a sweet vibe that's so chic.

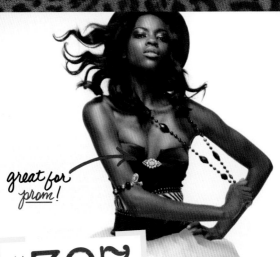

great for prom!

#307

adding a brooch

to your dress will draw attention to the nearest body part.

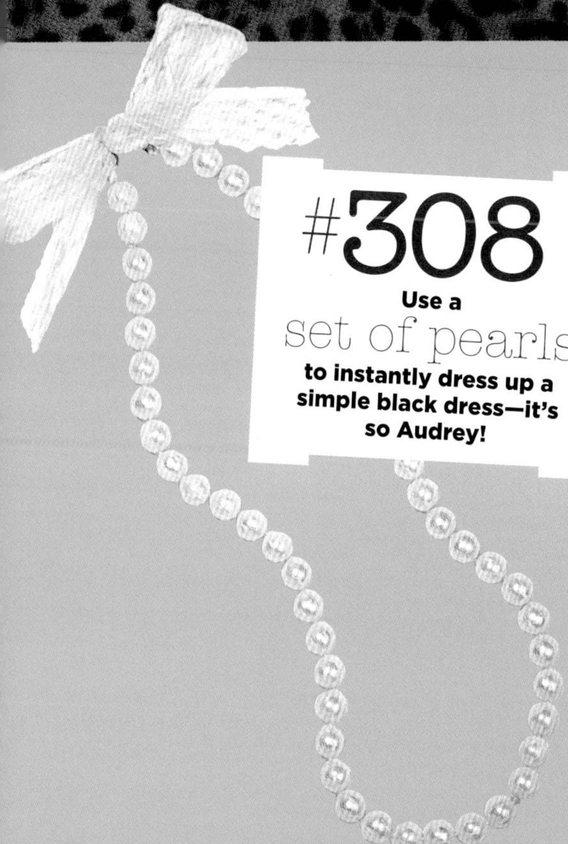

#308

Use a
set of pearls
to instantly dress up a
simple black dress—it's
so Audrey!

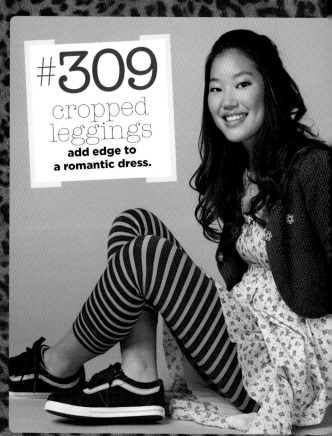

#309
cropped
leggings
**add edge to
a romantic dress.**

great for a <u>small</u> bust!

#310

A dress with a
gathered top
fills out your upper body.

great for
a _full_ bust!

#311

a fitted, high-cut tank

minimizes your bust but still shows off your figure.

#312

To survive
high heels,
**stick padded adhesive
shoe cushions
inside your shoes.**

great for prom!

#313

a metallic bag

adds a little bit of party flash to a basic jeans-and-top outfit.

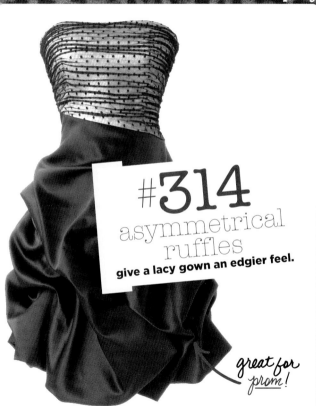

#314
asymmetrical
ruffles
give a lacy gown an edgier feel.

great for prom!

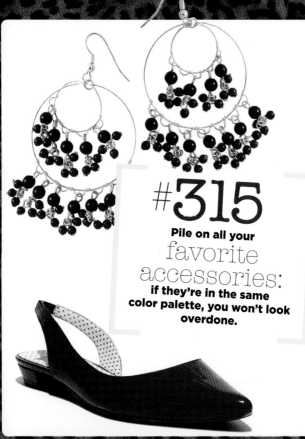

#315

Pile on all your

favorite

accessories:

**if they're in the same
color palette, you won't look
overdone.**

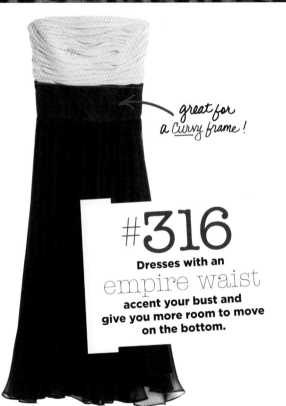

great for a curvy frame!

#316

Dresses with an
empire waist
accent your bust and give you more room to move on the bottom.

great for prom!

#317

When you try a wild
cut-out shape,
**stick with classic (and classy) black
and white so your look stays chic.**

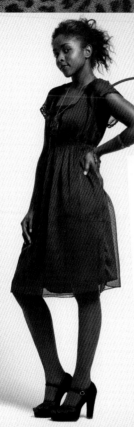

great for <u>petite</u> girls!

#318

If you want to add the illusion of height, try an outfit in

one solid color

to create a long, lean line.

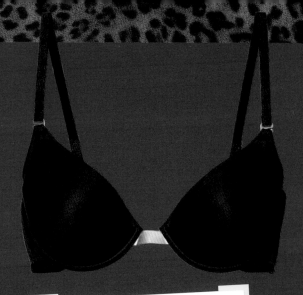

#319
leave your lacy
bras in the drawer when getting dressed up: Styles with lace or ribbon will only create lumps and bumps under clingy tops!

#320

Wipe a dime-size amount of petroleum jelly on your

patent-leather

shoes and rub in completely to give them a shiny, like-new finish.

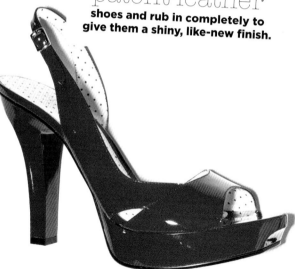

#321

A fun dress with a
big bow
is a party staple—you're like a pretty present all wrapped up!

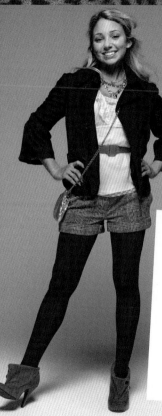

#322

**Style rules are
looser for a party
night—try**
textured
tights
**under shorts for
a change.**

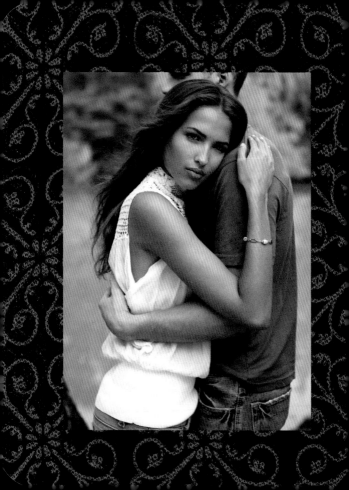

date

Whether it's a first date or a night out with your serious love, you want to look cute and confident—and just a bit flirty. Turn the page for sweet styles you (and he) will love.

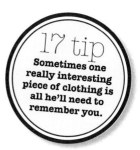

17 tip

Sometimes one really interesting piece of clothing is all he'll need to remember you.

#323

earthy jewelry

is a way to show off your personality when you wear it with a simple top.

#324
a fitted
blazer
**draws the eye to
a tiny waistline.**

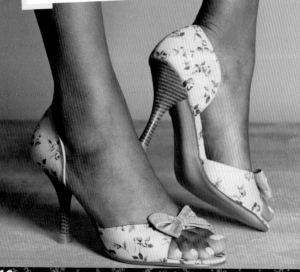

#325

peep-toe shoes

with pretty details like flowers and satin bows have a romantic vibe.

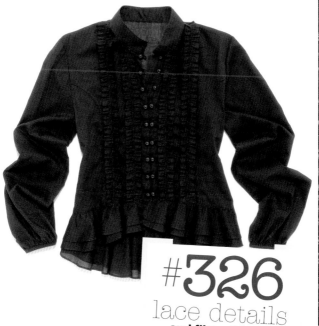

#326
lace details
**and flirty ribbons
make you look soft and
approachable.**

#327

Let a little

lace tank

peek out from under your jacket to look sweetly flirty.

#328

When your skirt is super short, wear lots of layers on top **to balance your look.**

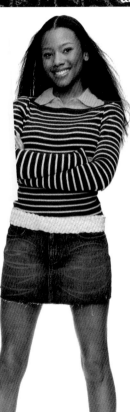

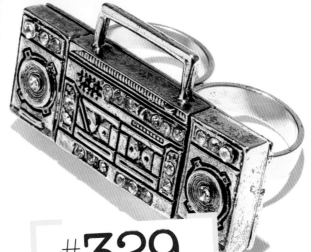

#329
a crazy piece
of jewelry
**shows your spontaneous,
fun-loving side.**

#330

Show off your
brightest shoes
by wearing capris!

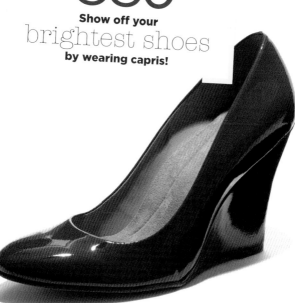

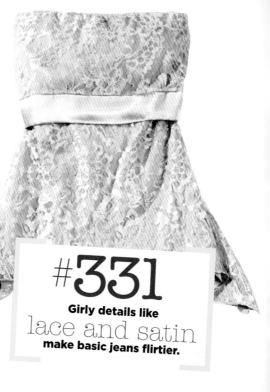

#331

Girly details like

lace and satin
make basic jeans flirtier.

#332

A cute sleeveless top paired with a

thick, cozy scarf

bares just the right amount of skin.

great for a _small_ bust !

#333

A lace-trimmed
V-neck dress
**subtly fills out
a petite upper body.**

#334
golden accents
give *every* look a glam vibe.

#335

an off-the-shoulder top

makes your upper body look broader (and your lower body look narrower)!

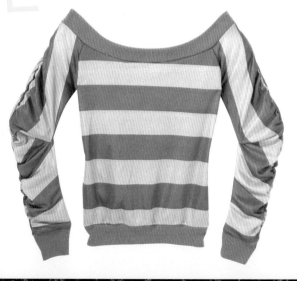

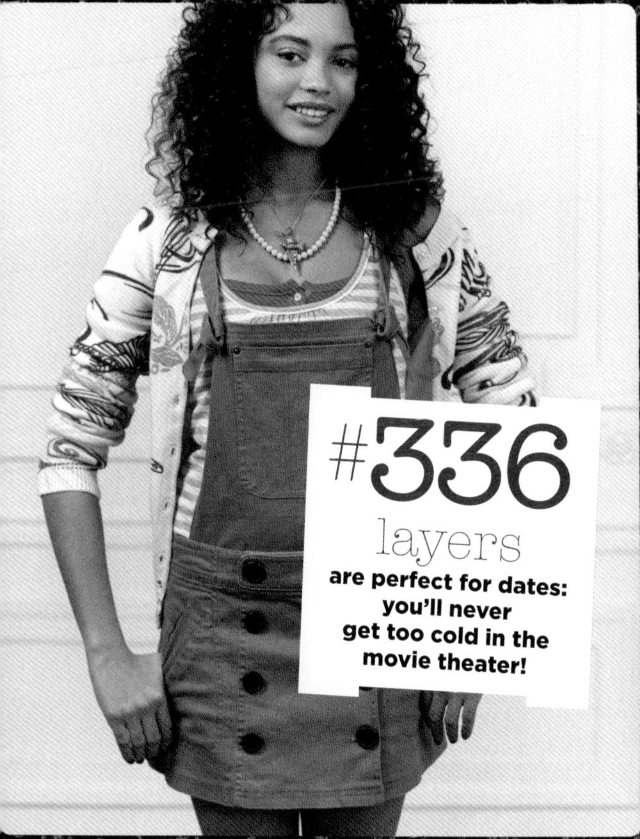

#336

layers

**are perfect for dates:
you'll never
get too cold in the
movie theater!**

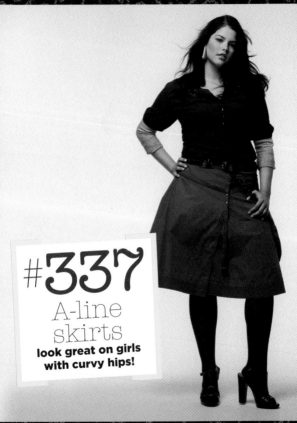

#337
A-line
skirts
**look great on girls
with curvy hips!**

#338
dark leggings
**under a dress
create a sleek silhouette.**

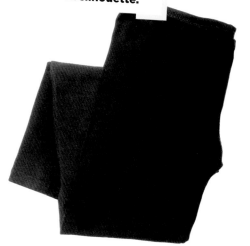

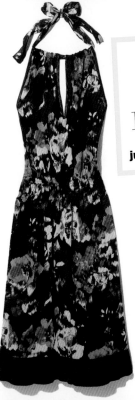

#339

Wear a sexy
keyhole top
**for a cute way to show
just a tiny bit of cleavage.**

#340

Pick a pair of

tailored jeans

long enough to wear with heels for a put-together look.

great for a *small* bust!

#341

a ruffle-
trimmed
**cami fills out
a smaller chest.**

#342

Bring just a touch of

va-va-voom

to your favorite look with a glittery scarf.

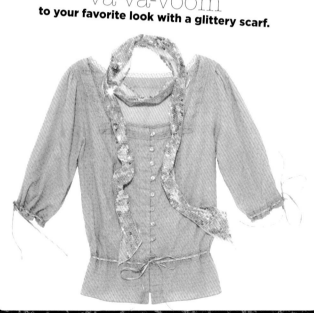

#343

Look for a mini that has subtle
embellishments—
they'll definitely catch his eye!

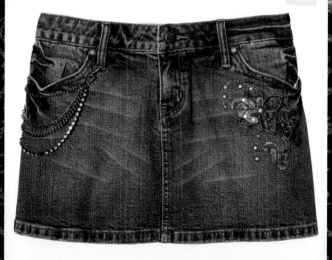

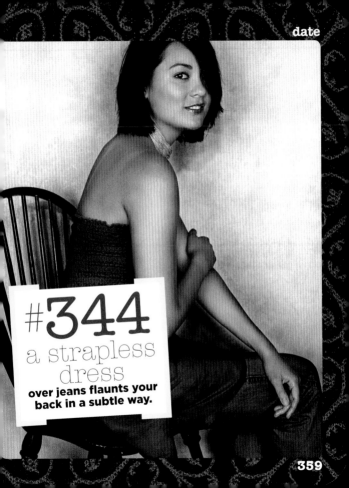

#344
a strapless
dress
**over jeans flaunts your
back in a subtle way.**

#345
a fitted
coat
looks trendy *and* has a slimming effect.

#346
a handkerchief hem
draws the eye to your sexy calves.

#347
halter
necks
**highlight a long neck
and graceful arms.**

#348

**Give a basic tee a fancier
look with a pretty**

sweater shrug.

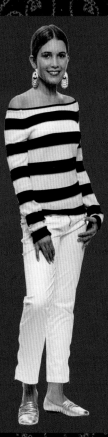

#349

When wearing an off-the-shoulder top, keep hair swept back and wear

dangling earrings

to show off your neckline.

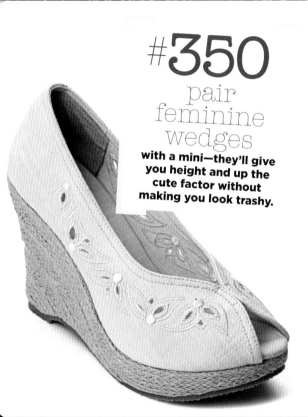

#350
pair feminine wedges

with a mini—they'll give you height and up the cute factor without making you look trashy.

#351

a slipdress

can be a great layering piece. Try it over a turtleneck and jeans or under a fitted blazer.

great for an hourglass shape!

#352
pick a headband
that contrasts with your hair color so it pops!

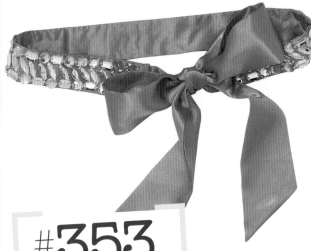

#353

a ribbon belt

draws tons of attention to your middle!

#354
lush-looking brocade
pieces will give you a romantic, Victorian look.

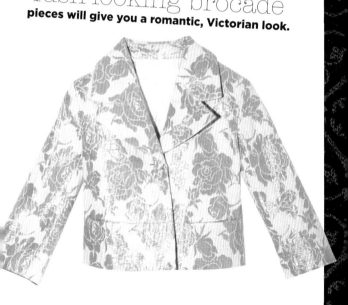

#355

Carry an
unusual bag
**to give a classic outfit an
unexpected, eclectic touch.**

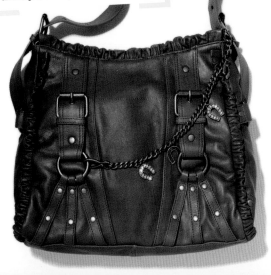

#356

A super-long
tunic
**doubles as a
short flirty dress!**

#357

Balance a

voluminous dress

by wearing a fitted tank underneath—it's a subtly sexy statement.

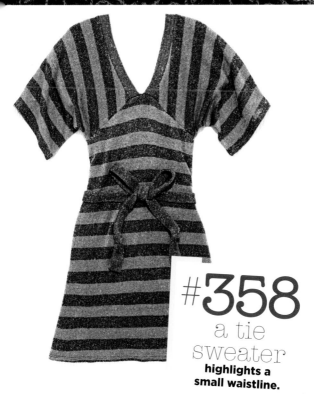

#358
a tie sweater
highlights a small waistline.

[#359

Slim jeans and
wedges
make legs look longer.

]

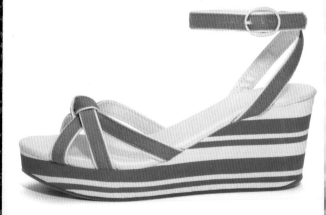

great for a <u>curvy</u> frame!

#360
a soft fabric
**like jersey knit
skims over any bulges
and feels comfy!**

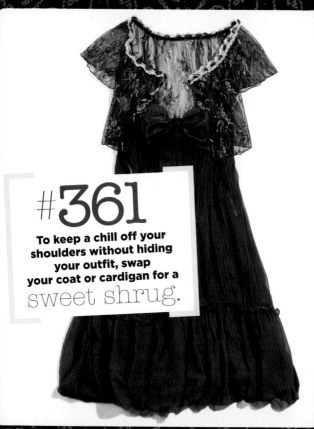

#361

To keep a chill off your shoulders without hiding your outfit, swap your coat or cardigan for a

sweet shrug.

#362
a heart-print top
looks adorably retro *and* sends a subtle message!

#363

Wear a

charm
necklace

**to add a dash of color to
a simple outfit.**

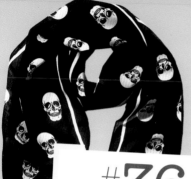

#364
a skull-patterned
scarf screams coolness.

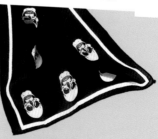

great for a small bust!

#365

A sweetheart neckline with gathering **fills out your bust.**

#366

a silky
dress

**layered under a
sporty jacket
combines a little
flirtation with a lot
of comfort.**

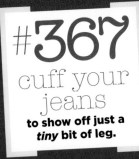

#367
cuff your jeans
to show off just a *tiny* bit of leg.

#368
cute flats
with skinny jeans are perfect!

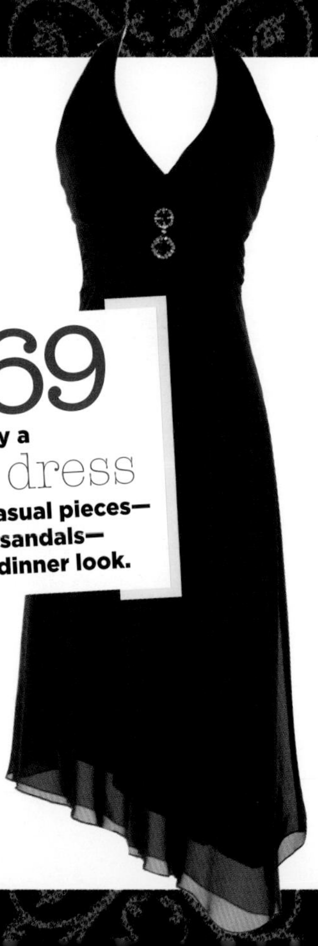

#369

Try a
glam dress
with more casual pieces—
like flat sandals—
for a chic dinner look.

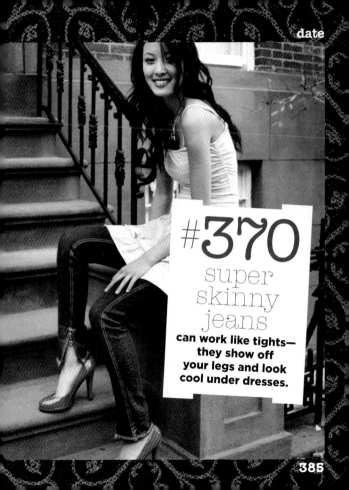

#370
super skinny jeans

can work like tights— they show off your legs and look cool under dresses.

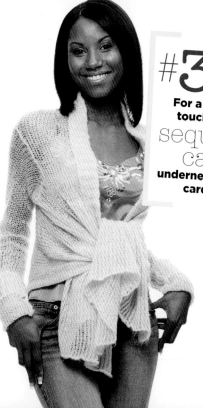

#371

For a feminine touch, wear a sequined cami **underneath a wrap cardigan.**

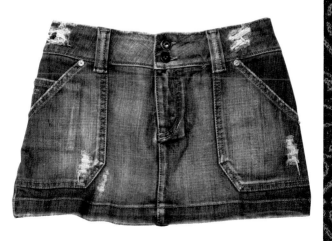

#372

a distressed
**denim mini has a laid-back,
"I'm low maintenance
but still cute" vibe.**

great for
an athletic
figure!

#373
an open-back top
is a dramatic way to show off a sculpted upper body.

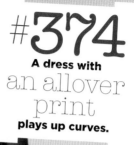

#374

A dress with
an allover print
plays up curves.

#375

Instead of matching your *shoes* to fit your outfit, make them contrast to show off your great taste!

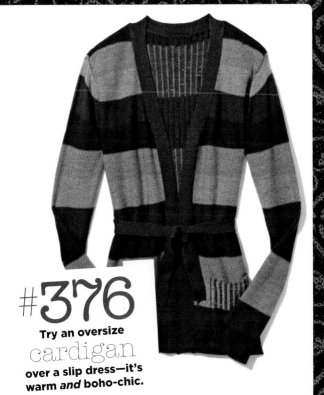

#376

Try an oversize *cardigan* **over a slip dress—it's warm** *and* **boho-chic.**

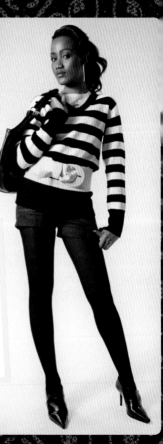

#377

dark
stockings

**and heels add a
sophisticated touch
to short shorts.**

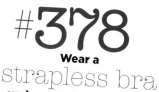

#378

Wear a

strapless bra

**under a slinky camisole—
letting your straps show on a
date is tacky.**

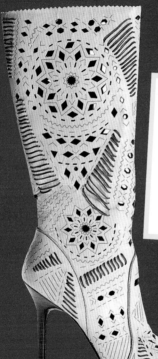

#379

wear
stiletto
boots
**with tucked-in jeans
to show them off!**

#380
a boxy jacket
becomes super-sexy with skinny pants.

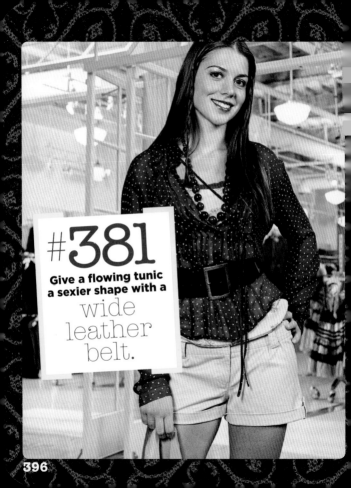

#381

Give a flowing tunic a sexier shape with a wide leather belt.

#382
High-heeled
ankle boots
**are a perfect
pair with skinny jeans.**

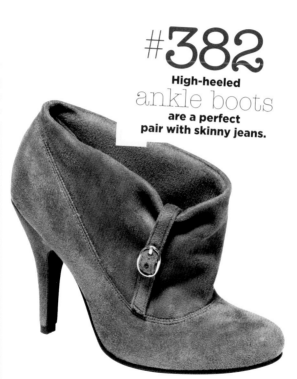

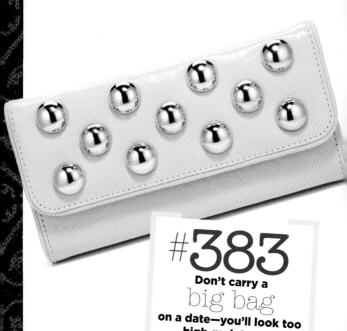

#383
Don't carry a
big bag
**on a date—you'll look too
high-maintence.
Keep it small and chic!**

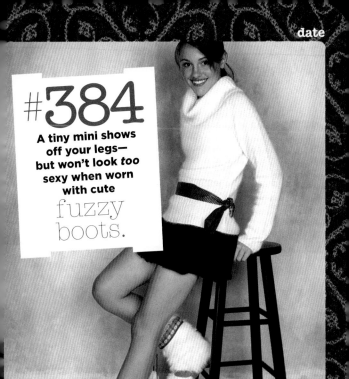

#384

A tiny mini shows off your legs— but won't look *too* sexy when worn with cute fuzzy boots.

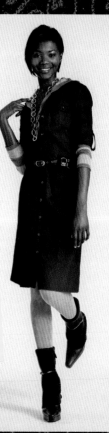

#385

colored hosiery

draws attention to your legs and makes them look shapelier.

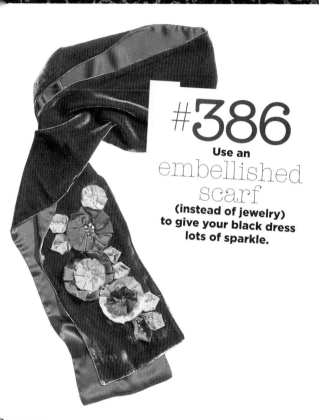

#386
Use an
*embellished
scarf*
**(instead of jewelry)
to give your black dress
lots of sparkle.**

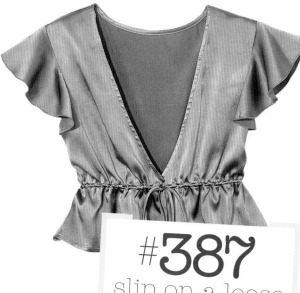

#387
slip on a loose shrug
to subtly cover your bust and play up your waist.

#388

Layered, chunky necklaces and

long, dramatic earrings

draw the eye up to your gorgeous face.

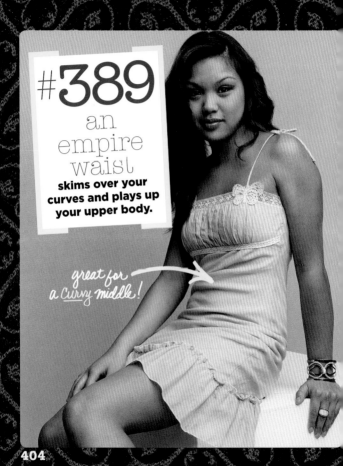

#389

an empire waist

skims over your curves and plays up your upper body.

great for a curvy middle!

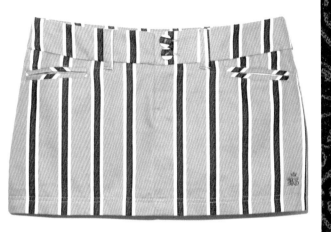

#390
a super-mini
works best with sneakers.

#391

a bright tank

underneath a sexy black-lace cami gives it a fun twist.

#392
animal prints
give off a sexy, spontaneous vibe.

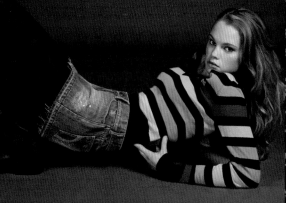

#393

opaque tights

**and rugged boots make a short
skirt cool, not skanky.**

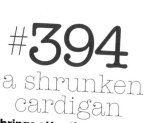

#394
a shrunken cardigan

brings attention to your waist—yet it doesn't bare anything at all!

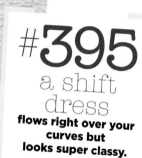

#395
a shift dress
flows right over your curves but looks super classy.

great for a curvy middle!

#396

A structured

velvet
blazer

is casual, rocker, and polished all at *once*!

#397

Give light, relaxed layers a nautical feel by tying a rope belt **just above your waist.**

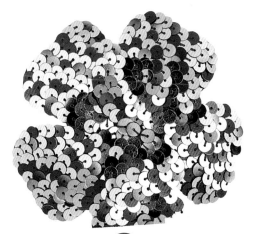

#398

**Personalize a simple dress by
pinning a vintage or**

sparkly brooch

**to the bustline—right
where the straps meet the dress.**

great for a <u>straight body</u>!

#399
a mini with soft pleats
gives boyish bodies a sexier look.

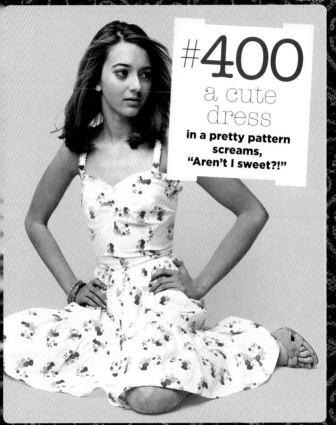

#400
a cute
dress

in a pretty pattern screams, "Aren't I sweet?!"

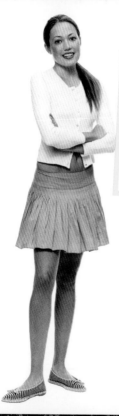

#401

To keep from showing too much skin, pair a hip-hugging miniskirt with a buttoned-up cardigan.

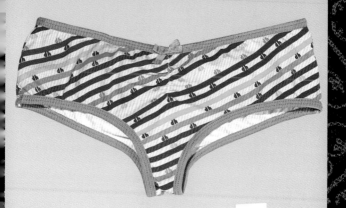

#402
hipster, boy-cut undies
**work great with low-cut jeans—
you won't show off your
butt whenever you sit down!**

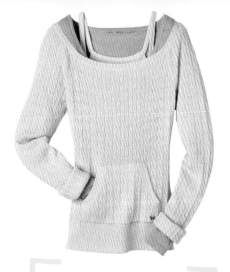

#403
put a cami
**underneath a
tunic to create a flirty look.**

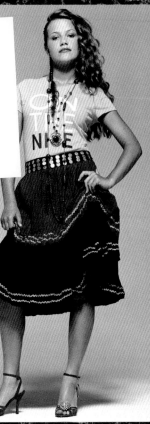

#404

A flowing skirt with a
decorated
waistband
**highlights
a small midsection.**

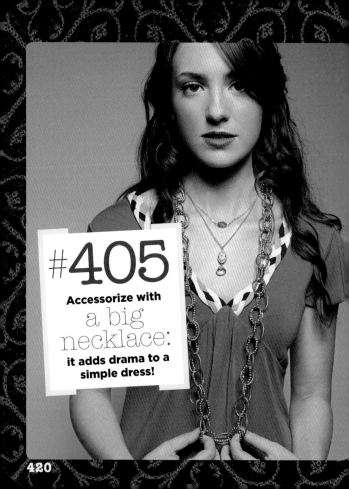

#405

Accessorize with
a big
necklace:
**it adds drama to a
simple dress!**

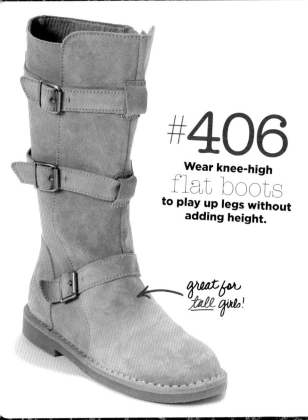

#406

Wear knee-high flat boots **to play up legs without adding height.**

great for <u>tall</u> girls!

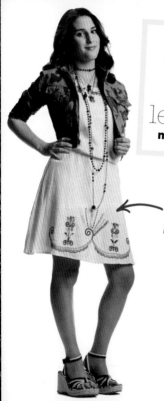

#407
a knee-length dress
makes legs look longer.

great for <u>petite</u> girls!

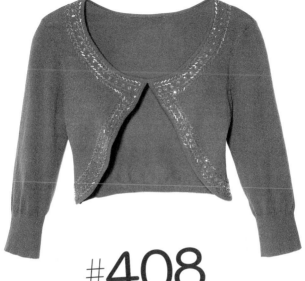

#408

Pair a black tee with a glittery
beaded shrug
for a sophisticated look.

#409

a wild
floral
design

**paired with colorful
shoes evokes the
carefree '70s—it's a
cool, fun statement.**

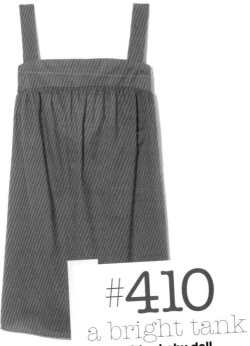

#410
a bright tank
**with a baby doll
cut looks great with leggings.**

great for an *hourglass* shape!

#411
a belted dress
shows off a tiny top half while hiding hips.

#412
Button a
sparkly cardigan
only at the top to show just a sliver of skin.

#413

Give a sweet dress a little edge with a

studded bag.

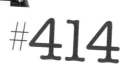

#414

For a more casual date, a
jumper
is cute and incredibly cool.

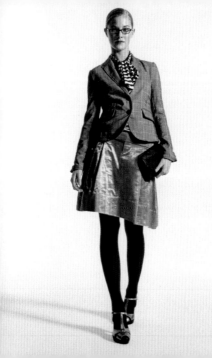

work

Who says work clothes have to be stuffy? Sophisticated and chic is key when you're getting dressed for your internship or job, so don't be afraid to add a unique touch or two to your buttoned-up look. This section is packed with practical tips.

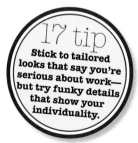

17 tip

Stick to tailored looks that say you're serious about work—but try funky details that show your individuality.

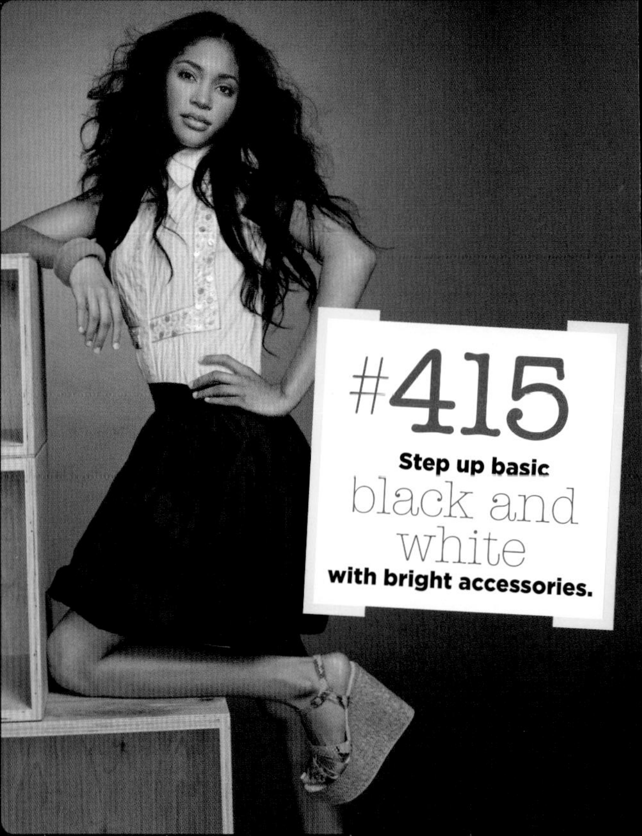

#415

Step up basic
black and
white
with bright accessories.

#416

a proper plaid

**can still be fun in a fitted jacket
(but totally cool for work).**

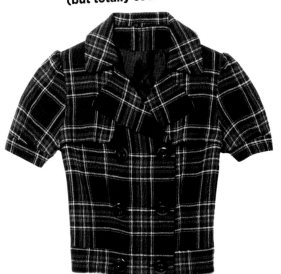

#417
a floaty white
sweater
**is delicate *and* demure over a
scoop-neck cotton top.**

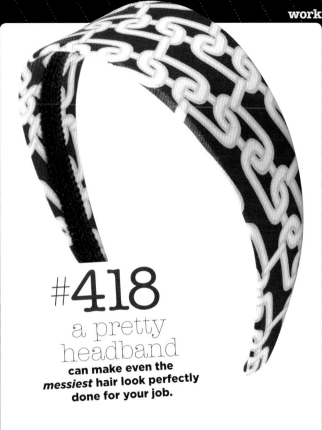

#418

a pretty headband

can make even the *messiest* hair look perfectly done for your job.

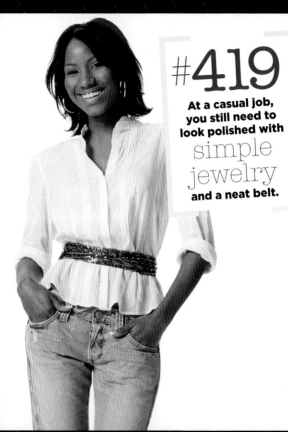

#419

At a casual job,
you still need to
look polished with
simple
jewelry
and a neat belt.

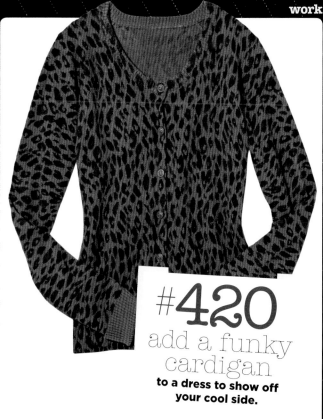

#420
add a funky cardigan
to a dress to show off your cool side.

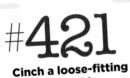

#421

Cinch a loose-fitting dress with a *ribbon* **for a cool, retro feel.**

#422
tuck khakis
into high boots for a look that's trendy but still neat.

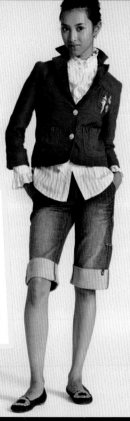

#423

blazers

always look professional—layer a soft blouse under one for a more feminine take.

#424
flared
trousers
**look sophisticated
and don't cling to
your curves.**

*great for
curvy hips
and thighs!*

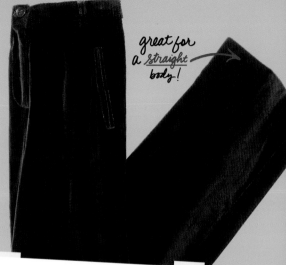

great for a *straight* body!

#425
wide-leg pants
make your body look curvier and they're always work-appropriate.

442

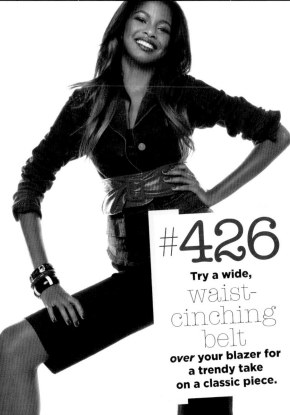

#426

Try a wide,
waist-cinching belt
***over* your blazer for
a trendy take
on a classic piece.**

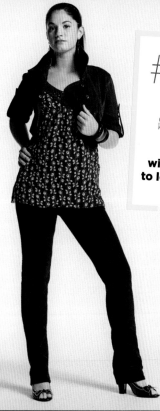

#427

Pair a

shruken jacket

with a long tunic top to look sophisticated— but still hot!

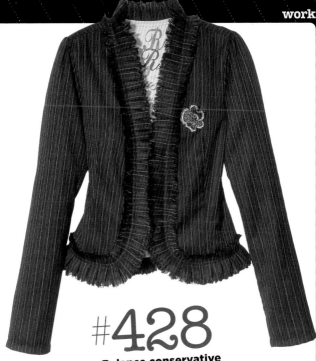

#428

Balance conservative
pinstripes
with a frilly brooch.

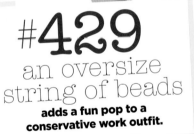

#429
an oversize
string of beads
**adds a fun pop to a
conservative work outfit.**

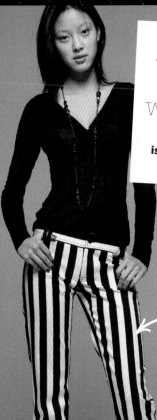

#430

One bold piece like

wide-striped
pants

**is all you need to stand
out at the job.**

*great for
curvy thighs!*

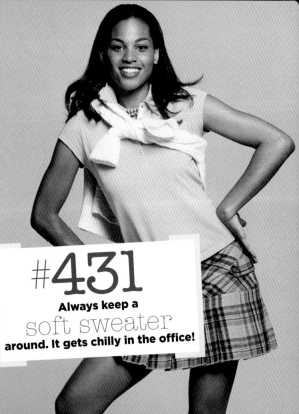

#431
Always keep a
soft sweater
around. It gets chilly in the office!

#432
a cropped blazer
lets you show off a cool belt.

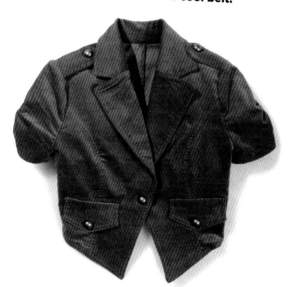

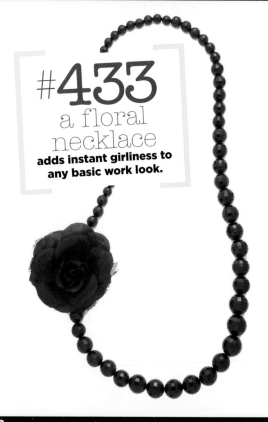

#433
a floral
necklace
**adds instant girliness to
any basic work look.**

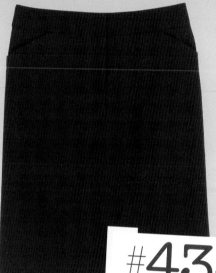

#434
a black
pencil skirt
**is a timeless staple
that always looks polished.**

#435

Be a little cheeky by wearing
your little
brother's tie.

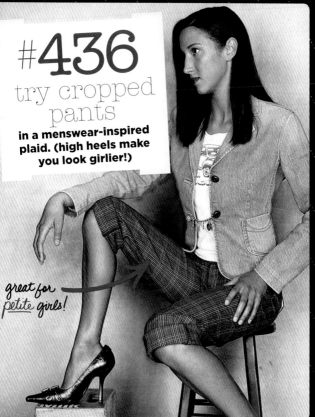

#436
try cropped pants

in a menswear-inspired plaid. (high heels make you look girlier!)

great for petite girls!

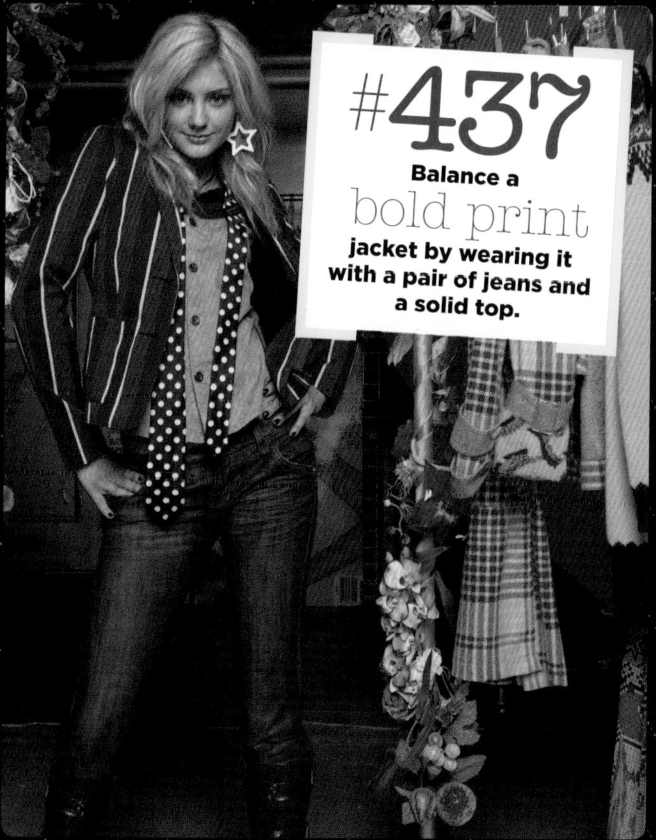

#437

Balance a
bold print
**jacket by wearing it
with a pair of jeans and
a solid top.**

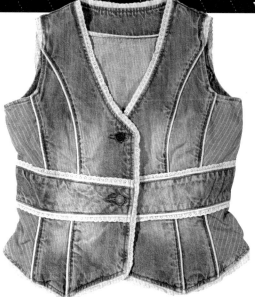

#438
dress up a denim vest
with a sweet skirt and work-appropriate flats.

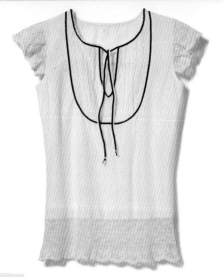

#439

a soft blouse
looks professional with a simple skirt.

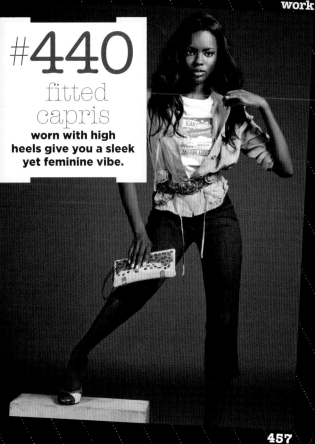

#440
fitted
capris
**worn with high
heels give you a sleek
yet feminine vibe.**

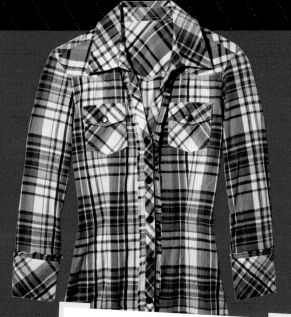

#441

For work, make sure a

button-down shirt

doesn't gap open over your bust!

#442

Style a
metallic
braided belt
**over a flowing floral dress
to play down its sweetness.**

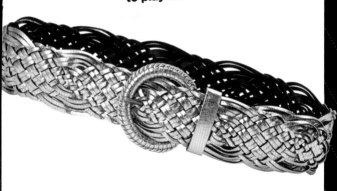

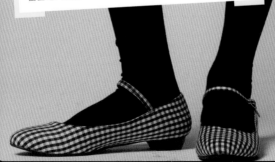

#443

Give your outfit a preppy twist with

houndstooth flats.

#444
a fun pendant
**lets your personality
shine through your work outfit.**

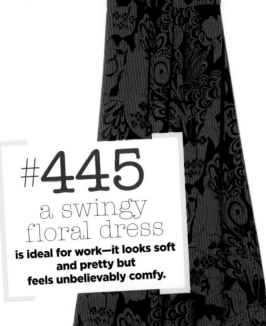

#445

a swingy floral dress

is ideal for work—it looks soft and pretty but feels unbelievably comfy.

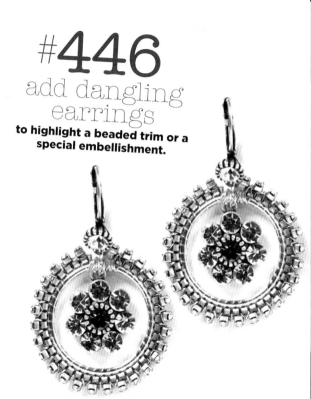

#446
add dangling
earrings
**to highlight a beaded trim or a
special embellishment.**

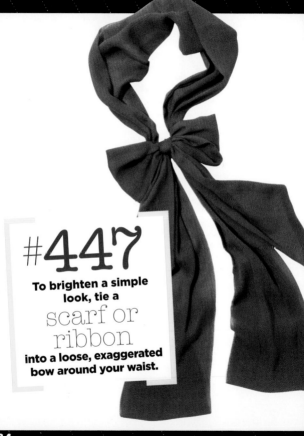

#447

To brighten a simple look, tie a scarf or ribbon **into a loose, exaggerated bow around your waist.**

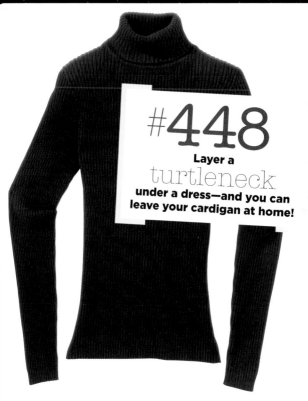

#448

Layer a

turtleneck

**under a dress—and you can
leave your cardigan at home!**

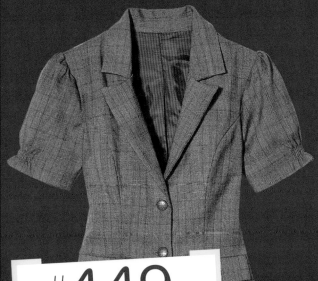

#449

Wear a

fitted jacket

buttoned up as a top—it's a fresh way to look pulled-together.

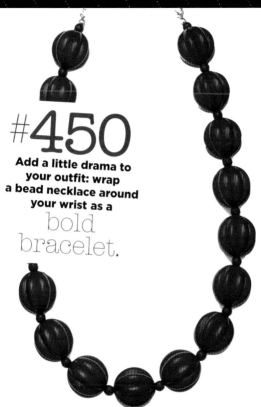

#450

Add a little drama to your outfit: wrap a bead necklace around your wrist as a bold bracelet.

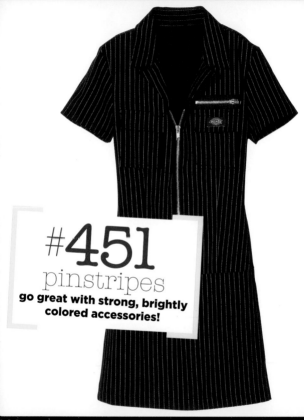

#451
pinstripes
**go great with strong, brightly
colored accessories!**

#452
a knee-
length skirt
balances super-long legs.

great for
tall girls!

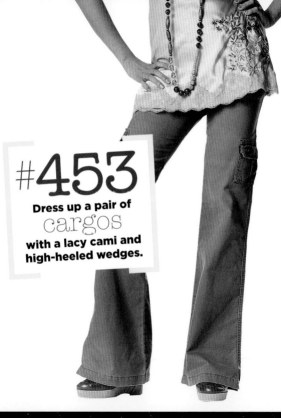

#453

Dress up a pair of
cargos
**with a lacy cami and
high-heeled wedges.**

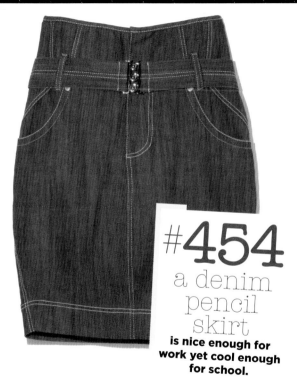

#454
a denim
pencil
skirt
**is nice enough for
work yet cool enough
for school.**

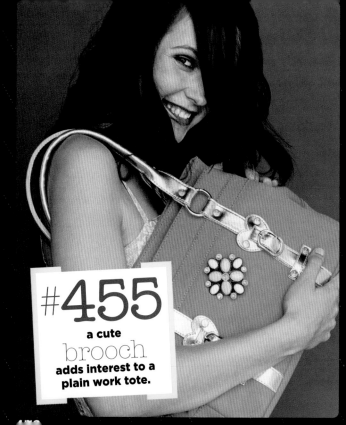

#455

a cute
brooch
adds interest to a
plain work tote.

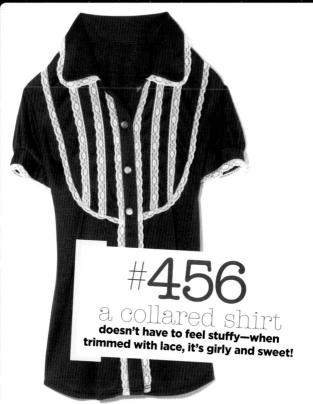

#456

a collared shirt

doesn't have to feel stuffy—when trimmed with lace, it's girly and sweet!

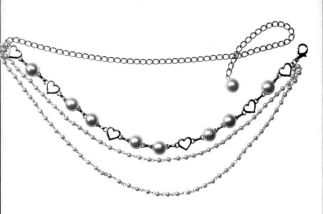

#457

Try pearls with a
hint of color
**(like pink)—it's a modern take on
an age-old classic.**

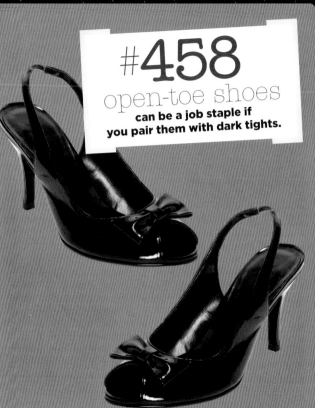

#458
open-toe shoes
**can be a job staple if
you pair them with dark tights.**

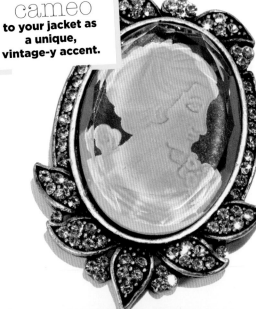

#459

Pin a classic *cameo* **to your jacket as a unique, vintage-y accent.**

#460

try one solid color
to streamline your hips and bust.

*great for
an hourglass
shape!* →

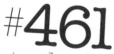

great for <u>petite</u> girls!

#461
a to-the-knee pleated skirt
creates a lean line, so your body looks taller.

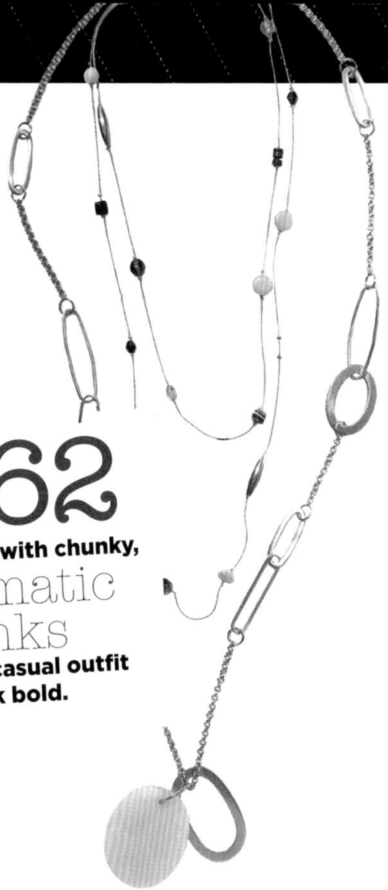

#462

A necklace with chunky,
dramatic
links
**makes a casual outfit
look bold.**

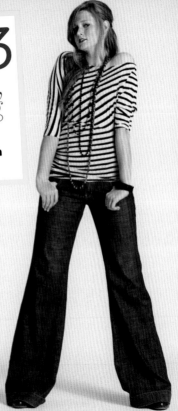

#463

flowing,
wide-leg
pants

**look best with a
fitted top.**

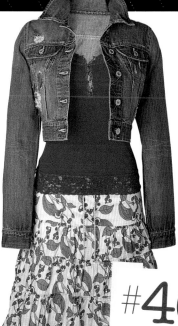

#464

a full skirt

that hits close to the knee draws the eye to your calves.

great for a curvy frame!

#465

Make a revealing

wrap-around dress

okay for your job—put a tee under it and a fitted blazer *over* it.

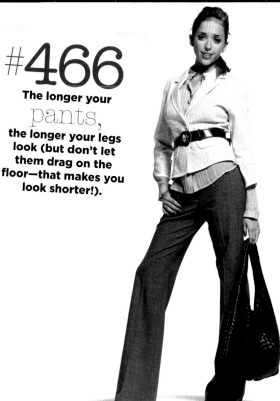

#466
The longer your
pants,
**the longer your legs
look (but don't let
them drag on the
floor—that makes you
look shorter!).**

#467

For the most comfort, buy

pointy-toe
shoes

**a half size bigger than usual.
This way, your
toes won't feel crammed In.**

#468

A bold
pattern
dress
can **work at your job—just tone it down with a solid cardigan.**

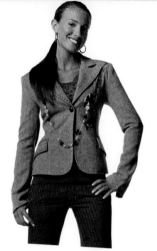

#469

mix and match

a cute blazer with pants–it's professional but has more personality than a stuffy suit.

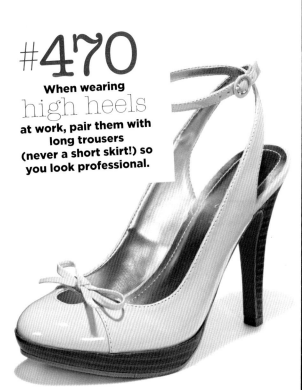

#470

When wearing
high heels
**at work, pair them with
long trousers
(never a short skirt!) so
you look professional.**

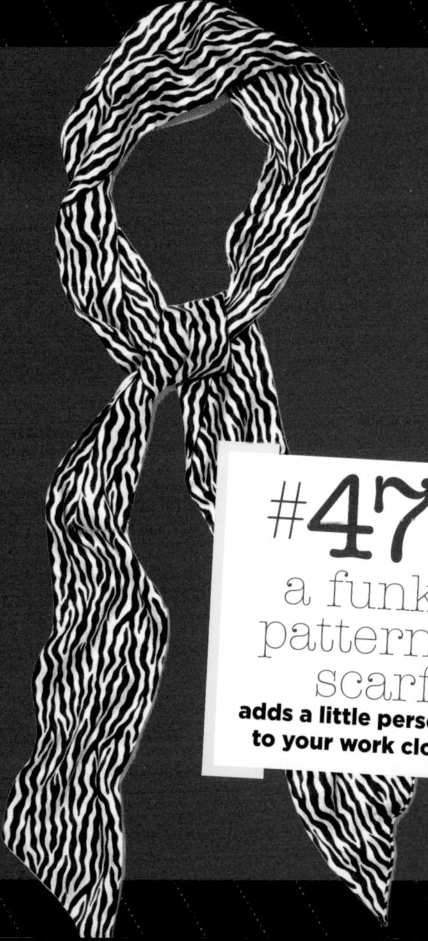

#471

a funky,
patterned
scarf
**adds a little personality
to your work clothes.**

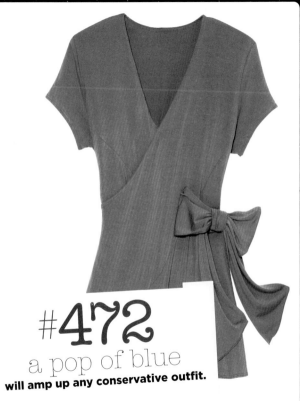

#472
a pop of blue
will amp up any conservative outfit.

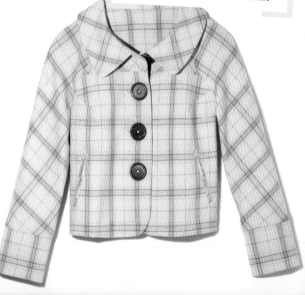

#473

a boxy blazer

has super-chic '60s flair.

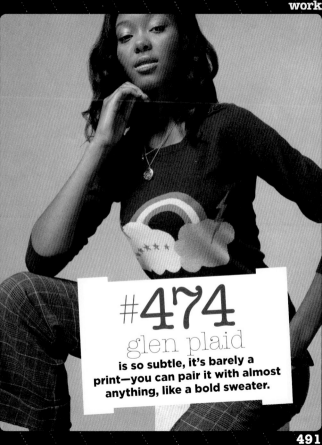

#474
glen plaid
is so subtle, it's barely a print—you can pair it with almost anything, like a bold sweater.

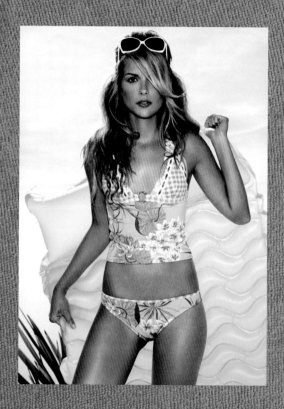

pool

It's hard for anyone to turn down poolside fun or a day at the beach with friends. Make the most of it by looking *hot* in your swim gear! Check out this chapter for the styles and fits that suit you best.

17 tip

Wearing the right suit for your body type will help you feel confident—so you'll have more fun!

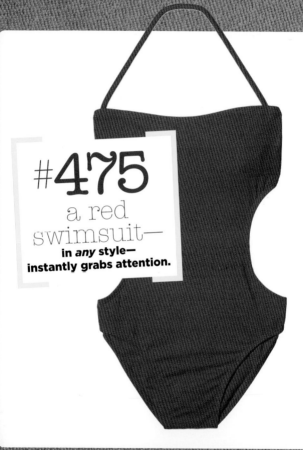

#475

a red
swimsuit—
in *any* style—
instantly grabs attention.

#476
a bandeau top
means no weird tan lines.

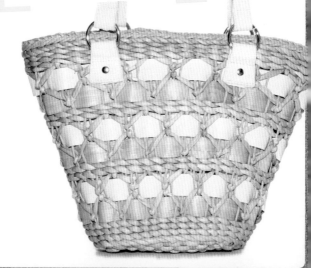

#477

a straw bag

with leather trim is casual enough for the beach but pretty enough for going out.

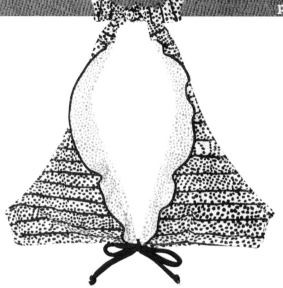

#478

a tie-front top

creates subtle cleavage.

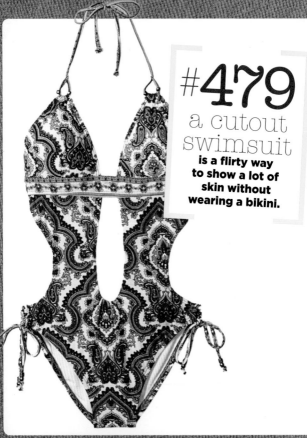

#479

a cutout swimsuit

is a flirty way to show a lot of skin without wearing a bikini.

#480
underwire
**creates shaping and coverage
that feels like your favorite bra.**

#481
string bottoms
actually have a narrowing effect on your butt—seriously!

great for a curvy butt!

billabong

#482

a tube dress
**is easy to slip over a bikini
and to roll into your bag.**

#483
a high-cut suit
makes legs look longer.

great for petite girls!

#484
boy-cut shorts
create the illusion of curvier hips.

great for a straight figure!

#485

a high-cut
string bottom

**works on everyone's hips—
it's completely adjustable!**

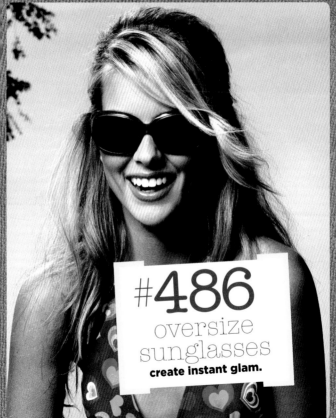

#486
oversize
sunglasses
create instant glam.

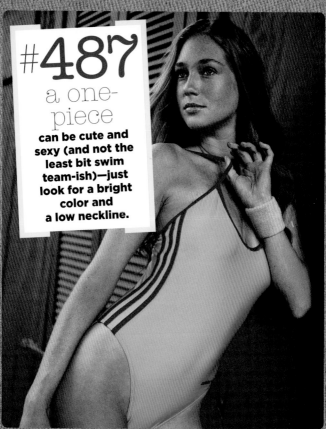

#487

a one-piece

can be cute and sexy (and not the least bit swim team-ish)—just look for a bright color and a low neckline.

#488

Tie your

string bikini bottoms

high on your hip—it will visually lengthen your legs (instead of cutting them off in an unflattering way).

#489

a graphic pair
of shorts

look fun with a solid bathing suit.

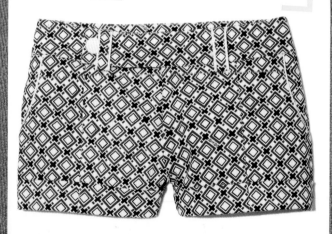

#490
horizontal stripes
fill you out and give the look of curves.

#491
A ruffled
skirtini
adds some volume to your backside.

great for a small butt!

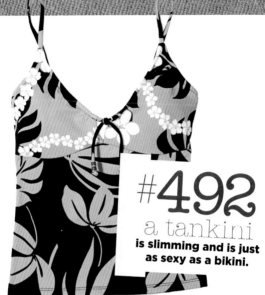

#492

a tankini

is slimming and is just as sexy as a bikini.

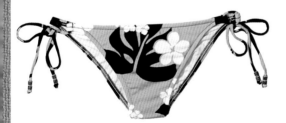

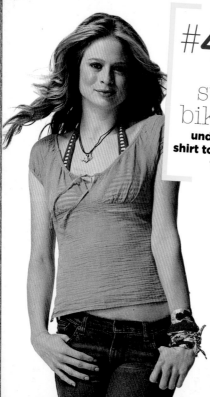

#493

Layer a

striped
bikini top

**under your solid
shirt to go from beach
to street.**

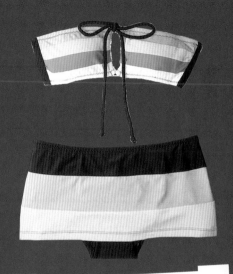

#494
a swim skirt
makes every body look narrower.

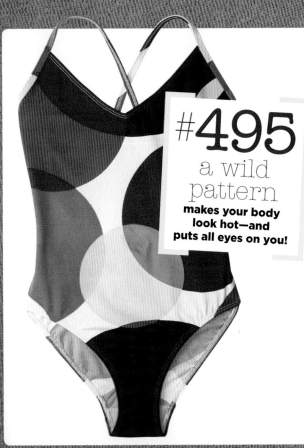

#495

a wild
pattern

**makes your body
look hot—and
puts all eyes on you!**

great for
a _full_ bust!

#496
halter tops
**offer the best support
while giving
you a flattering shape.**

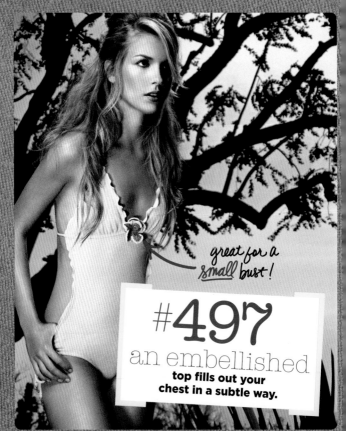

great for a _small_ bust!

#497

an embellished
top fills out your chest in a subtle way.

#498

aviator
sunglasses

**have a timeless style and give
off a cool retro vibe.**

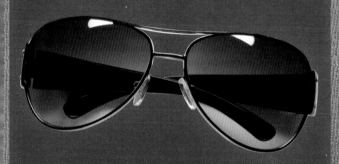

#499

Create a cute
waistband
**by letting your swimsuit
bottoms peek out
from underneath jeans.**

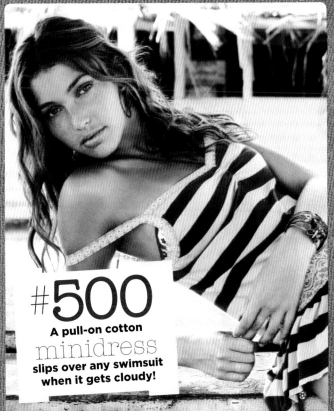

#500

A pull-on cotton

minidress

slips over any swimsuit when it gets cloudy!

index

photos